Copyright 1988
NewLifestyle Books

Printed in the United States of America

Family Health Publications
8777 E. Musgrove Hwy.
Sunfield, MI. 48890

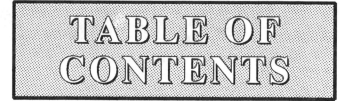

iv

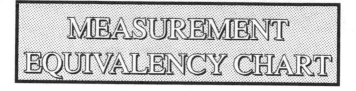

MEASUREMENT EQUIVALENCY CHART

1 gram = 0.03527 oz.   16 ounces = 1 pound
1 kilogram = 2.2046 lbs.   1 cup = 8 ounces
1 oz. = 28.35 grams   1 tablespoonful = 1 fl. ounce
1 lb. = .4536 kilograms   16 tablespoonsful = 1 cupful
           1 liter = 1.06 quarts liquid, 0.9 qt. dry
           3 teaspoonsful = 1 tablespoonful
16 drams = 1 ounce   1 tablespoonful = 1/2 ounce
           1 large wine glass = 2 ounces
           4 tablespoons flour = 1 ounce
           60 drops = 1 teaspoonful
           1 cup cornmeal = 5 ounces

1 cup bread crumbs (stale) = 2 ounces (1 cup of charcoal
       powder approximately the same weight)

           2 cups = 1 pint = 0.473 liters
           2 pints = 1 quart = 0.946 liters
           4 quarts = 1 gallon = 3.785 liters

       British dry quart = 1.032 U.S. dry quarts

10 milliliters = 1 centiliter = .338 fluid ounce
10 centiliters = 1 deciliter = 3.38 fluid ounces
10 deciliters = 1 liter = 1.0567 liquid quarts or .9081 dry quart
10 liters = 1 decaliter = 2.64 gallons or 2.838 bushels

CHAPTER 1

DIVINE PROVISION
MADE FOR HEALING

The forest...shadowy timeless place of towering trees and invisible rustlings; of hushed secrets whispered by the voiceless wind, its muteness made vocal through the ancient songs of a thousand warbler and thrush generations. Below, on the damp forest floor, lie strewn the long discarded foliage-garments of many summers past, together with the decomposing remains of former forest titans, brought low by storm, wind or age. Within a few short years, scattered mounds of spongy humus will alone mark their final resting place; that and nothing more. Thus life begets life and the forest goes on.

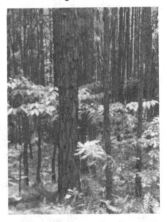

But something even more remarkable has taken place in this forest. Amidst the scrub and trailing vines lies the blackened hulk of another tree. Long ago it ceased to answer the awakening call of Spring; far longer than so many others now resting beneath the shadows. Little remains of them to give evidence a congregation in living green once stretched leafy branches heavenward here. So why does this charred tree remain and not itself go the way of all the others? Perhaps we have stumbled upon one of the very first wonders in the wonder of charcoal.

THE WONDER OF CHARCOAL

When wood is left on the ground, it begins to deteriorate immediately. If, however, a fire burns across the forest, wood is charred, retarding the deterioration process. Pieces of charred wood remain years longer than wood of the same size and type not in a charred condition. Charcoal, therefore, is simply charred wood. Not only does the charring process retard the deterioration of plant-life, but this end product, charcoal, has special

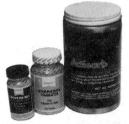 properties making it peculiarly useful in the human experience, its position being unfilled by any known substitute in industry, chemistry, toxicology, and the military.

Even traditional medicine has rediscovered the unparalleled properties of charcoal. As you read this book, you will learn more about the property of chemical attraction that charcoal possesses. We have found it able to take up toxic gases, disease germs, fluid toxic wastes or heavy metals. It is indeed a miracle substance.

EQUIPMENT AND SUPPLIES FOR HEALING

When we study human pathology (anatomy and function gone wrong), we find that certain mechanisms have been established for healing. We are able to recover from infectious diseases, nutritional deficiencies, fatigue, and injuries because of these "built-in features". A system is also provided for the cleansing of waste products or toxic exposures.

Psychological healing occurs in the form of forgetting,

a process well designed and so necessary in human experience. Additionally, healing is accomplished by our personal discipline and self-denial, exercise, fresh air, sunshine and food. With all else we have been created with, it would be strange indeed if nature did not provide a cleansing agent such as charcoal.

If there is anything evident from the study of nature, human physiology, and the history of mankind, it is that a loving, all-wise Creator has made provision for our every need. When we study human anatomy, we recognize that nothing is incomplete nor is anything missing from our anatomical structure that would be needful in carrying out every function of the body or mind. As we came from the hand of the Creator, "God saw everything...and...it was very good." We read with awe and great interest of the provision for a Saviour to give victory over sin. In the brain we see the neuronal pathways designed to form habits, and those used to inhibit habits. The mechanisms available to change a pattern of behavior are quite elaborate. We marvel that normal anatomy has been designed so well.

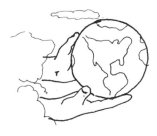

Many different provisions are made for healing and cleansing the body. Heat causes a certain physiologic response and stimulates impulses which go to the brain. Cold can have a similar influence. Pressure, massage, manipulation, and altering the position of various body parts all have a powerful influence to bring about healing. In every area we study, we see the hand of the divine Creator making provision for the body, its convenience, its smooth and trouble-free operation without conscious awareness of body parts, and an obvious provision for it to function eternally! That it does not do so is not the fault

3

of the Creator, but the influence of evil which arose as a result of a deliberate choice by intelligent beings even after experience with the goodness of the Creator--a choice that has brought immeasurable pain and discomfort to heaven and earth, and consternation to intelligent beings elsewhere in the universe.

CHAPTER 2

HOW CHARCOAL WORKS

SURVIVAL OF THE FITTEST REMEDIES

Charcoal has been used as a folk remedy as far back as recorded history. North American Indians used charcoal for the treatment of gas pains long before our forefathers came to this continent.

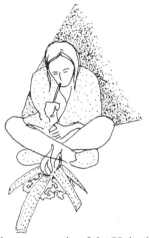

Homeopathic physicians have used charcoal throughout the world for more than 200 years. Carbo animalis (animal charcoal) and carbo vegetabilis (wood charcoal) have been carried in the homeopathic pharmacopoeia of the United States with the description that these substances have "marked absorptive power of gases."

Charcoal has been marketed by Rorer for many years in the prescription drug Chardonna, comprised of phenobarbital, belladonna extract and activated charcoal.[1] It has been used in the treatment of "nervous indigestion, gastritis, and flatulence." Charcoal is rated in Category I (safe and effective) status by the FDA for acute toxic poisoning.[2] Charcoal has been an official remedy in the United States for at least 100 years, and was eliminated from the U.S. Pharmacopoeia about 1950, not because it was ineffective, but because of its general disuse in American medicine following the phenomenal growth of the drug industry.

The light and fluffy black powder of charcoal has been used as a officially recognized antidote since the 19th century. It is easy to make by a destructive distillation of organic materials such as wood pulp, petroleum coke, coals, peat, sawdust, wood char, papermill waste, bone, and coconut shells. Any kind of wood such as willow, eucalyptus, pine, oak, and others are adequate sources of wood charcoal. Charcoals made from vegetable materials such as wood and coal contain about 90% carbon whereas bone charcoal contains about 11% carbon, 9% calcium carbonate, and 78% calcium phosphate.

PROPERTIES OF CHARCOAL

Certain electrostatic properties develop in activated charcoal during production which favor the binding of most poisons. When the gases, resins, proteins, fats, etc., in wood are burned out, the heat generated and the change in chemistry causes the development of a charge on the charcoal granule which attracts most poisonous substances.

Nobody has fully understood the mechanism by which charcoal works, from either a physical or chemical standpoint. The capillary attraction is felt to be one mechanism, the electrostatic forces another, and perhaps other forces are also involved.

Charred toast and other scorched food in the kitchen are not healthful, however. They are not charcoal. These represent charred protein, fats, carbohydrates, and mineral salts, the very parts burned away in charcoal, leaving only charred cellulose. The skeletal structure remaining in true charcoal is inert, whereas the remaining substances 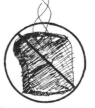 in charred food can react unhealthfully with the body, and even act as cancer-producing agents.

Activated charcoal is produced from the controlled burning of wood or bone which is then subjected to the action of an oxidizing gas such as steam or air at elevated temperatures. This process enhances the adsorptive power of charcoal by developing an extensive network of fine pores in the material. The activation process was not invented until after the turn of the 20th century, but charcoal was already recognized as a useful healing agent even though only regular charcoal was then in use. Following activation of charcoal with pressurized steam or strong acid, the surface area of one cubic centimeter is 1000 square meters! This expanded surface is due to the fact that charcoal particles have thousands of crevices, pits, grooves, and holes which, when opened out, make quite a large surface area.

The physical and chemical properties from the original material, and the condition of the carbonization process, 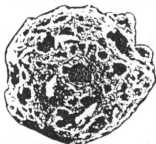 determine the properties of charcoal. The temperature of carbonization is about 600 degrees C. A hot blaze is maintained for one hour and then reduced to drop the temperature to 100-150 degrees C. by leaning the air which is maintained for days (or only hours if not very wet). Distillation then begins and the temperature rises to 600-700 degrees C. Kilns are closed during this process.

Tropical forests that have little marketable timber, make good charcoal woods--acacia, pinus, hardwoods, eucalyptus and others. Twenty to 30% of the dry weight of wood will represent the yield of charcoal, and about 50% of the volume of wood. Moisture content varies from 1-16%, volatile materials from 7-30%.

Retorts yield 25-30% more charcoal than kilns. They have slow carbonization at reduced temperatures giving a higher yield. The yield is greater when wood is cut to

7

uniform size and packed tightly in the retort. In making charcoal, oxygen is taken up rapidly the first few hours after carbonization has ceased. Spontaneous combustion is possible at this point. One might wonder if this taking up of oxygen, perhaps the unstable ionized form, is one explanation for the remarkable adsorptive property of charcoal. Debarking trees before igniting makes a cleaner and denser final product of charcoal. In 1970, the price was $477.00 per ton for wood charcoal and $100.00 per ton for coconut charcoal.[3]

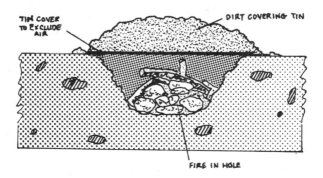

TIN COVER TO EXCLUDE AIR

DIRT COVERING TIN

FIRE IN HOLE

AVAILABILITY

Charcoal is readily available through commercial channels, but can also be made at home. When making your own charcoal, put pieces of wood in a fireplace or grill, char the wood well, then cut the charred portions from the wood with a sharp knife or machete, grind in a blender to a fine powder and use quite generously in the dosage schedules we recommend. This kind of charcoal must be used in about three to four times larger dosage than the activated charcoal. The ultimate in making your own charcoal begins with a wood fire out of doors. After the wood is burning brightly, it should be covered with a large piece of tin with dirt piled over the tin to make a dome to exclude air. As the heat continues to burn the wood with decreased oxygen, the soft parts of wood are

8

burned out first and the hard parts remain, making a good grade of charcoal. The charred parts of the wood should then be pounded to coarse granules in a cloth bag and ground in a blender to pulverize to a fine powder.

Commercial tablets are not as concentrated as charcoal capsules or the charcoal powder, being less effective by about half. In one study, humans took pulverized charcoal powder and prevented absorption of a drug by 73%. Those taking charcoal tablets were able to prevent absorption by only 48%, or roughly half. Tablets are made from regular charcoal and the pulverized powder is usually activated. Also about one-quarter of the tablet is starch material and other substances used to hold the tablets together. For tablets, chewing well is essential before swallowing to increase their effectiveness.

Briquettes for grilling food are not safe sources for either external or internal use, as various fillers and chemicals are applied to hold the charcoal together and to insure rapid igniting.

GENERAL NON-MEDICAL
USES OF CHARCOAL

Fuel savings in blast furnaces.
Soot clearance
Foundry work
Top dressings for gardens, bowling greens and lawns
Potting and bedding compounds
Prevention of water pollution
Sweeteners of the soil, mulch
Fertilizer and insecticide for roses
Water filter
Adsorption of pesticides and herbicides

CHAPTER 3

BLACK AND MESSY

INTRODUCTION

Many old-fashioned remedies have gone the way of homemade vegetable soup and push lawn mowers; not because they were undesirable or ineffective, but because there was an art required for their management, and an extra amount of labor involved in seeing the final results. Most people are unwilling to make the effort. *Such attitudes should be banished.* Knowledge and skill should be acquired to effectively use these valuable healing tools.

Every private home should have charcoal on hand as a ready antidote for poisoning, as a cleansing agent in infections, as a de-odorizer, and as the treatment of choice in diarrhea, nausea and vomiting, and many intestinal infections. Charcoal is harmless 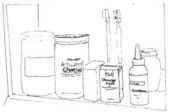 when ingested even in large quantities, or when inhaled in small quantities, and there are no ill effects when it comes in contact with the skin.

Because charcoal can pack molecules of ammonia gas into its crevices, it can attract and hold 80 quarts of ammonia gas per one quart of pulverized charcoal! This process is called adsorption, or attaching onto rather than taking into as in absorption. In 1773, Scheele made an experiment with charcoal in which a gas was trapped in an inverted tube with charcoal, the lower end of the tube being submerged in a container of mercury. As the gas was adsorbed by the charcoal, a vacuum appeared in the tube and sucked the mercury up into the tube. Pharmacist P.F. Touery, in 1831, making a demonstration of the effectiveness of charcoal before the French Academy of Medicine, survived after swallowing 15 grams of strychnine (ten times the lethal dose) and an equal amount of charcoal--about three tablespoonsful.

CHARCOAL DOSAGE

Although we have seen no problems with long-term use, as with all "treatments" we recommend that they be taken only as needed for acute conditions. Charcoal should not be taken regularly over a long period unless a serious long-term problem exists, such as gas and odors in colostomy and ileostomy patients. Occasionally someone will take a small dosage of charcoal on a regular basis as a prophylaxis or problem-preventer. If at all possible, it would be best to eliminate the toxic, infectious, or injurious agent rather than taking charcoal on a regular basis to counteract it. The reasons are several: 1) a dependency usually develops on a remedy where a maintenance program should be instituted; 2) the small possibility of interfering with nutrient balance; 3) the small expense and trouble, diverting money and time which should be used in more lofty pursuits.

There is still a marketing barrier because of unfamiliarity with handling the substance itself, and unfamiliarity with the amazing effectiveness of charcoal in many situations. The medical research done since 1970 is going far to rectify this situation. Even doctors have been unfamiliar with charcoal until recently.

Charcoal can be purchased as a powder, charcoal suspension in water, charcoal paste, tablets and capsules. The activated capsules are roughly twice as potent as the tablets. Drugstores or health food stores often carry charcoal. The oral dosage is one tablespoon of powder stirred into a small amount of water. Four capsules of activated charcoal represent about one tablespoonful, or eight tablets of regular charcoal. The dosage should be taken other than at mealtimes, as food tends to interfere with the adsorptive quality of charcoal. If charcoal is to be taken throughout the day, the best schedule is upon arising, midway between breakfast and lunch, midway between lunch and supper, and at bedtime. Food interferes with its best action.

There has been some discussion as to whether food and partially split derivatives of food, digestive enzymes, and various secretions usually found in the gastrointestinal tract would inhibit adsorption of drugs or poisons by charcoal. It has been found that there is approximately a 50% reduction in effectiveness when the stomach is filled. After heavy fat ingestion, bile reduces the adsorptive capabilities of charcoal by 30%, and duodenal juice causes a very minor reduction in effectiveness. When a poison is ingested while food is still in the stomach, to be on the safe side, we recommend approximately eight to ten times the estimated weight of the poison as the dosage of charcoal. Finely powdered charcoal can get to the surface of toxins better than coarsely powdered charcoal, and therefore should be used for best results. **For a quick ready reference on dosages, see the chart at the end of Chapter 5**.

A very sensitive person may occasionally feel a bit of irritation of the stomach with the use of charcoal. Another often unwanted action of charcoal is the prolonging of the transit time. Neither of these effects is really a contraindication to the use of charcoal, and can usually be avoided or treated by simply drinking several glasses of water. Allergies to charcoal have not been reported. Charcoal is inexpensive, harmless, and easily used. It is readily available through commercial channels, and can be made at home.

METHODS OF MAKING AND APPLYING
THE CHARCOAL COMPRESS

A charcoal compress for a large area such as the abdomen or a knee joint can be made as follows: three tablespoons of cornstarch or flax seed ground in a blender or seed mill and mixed with one to three tablespoons of pulverized charcoal. Stir into one cup of water, set aside for 10 to 20 minutes or heat slightly to thicken.

Spread the thickened mixture on a disposable (from the pharmacy) 15 x 20 inch bed underpad after cutting the thin fabric outer sheet around the edge on two sides with scissors. Spread the charcoal mixture about 1/4 inch thick over every bit of the pocket formed by opening up the underpad, reseal with masking tape, and the compress is made. Fasten it in place with a large bandage such as a towel of appropriate size which is pinned snugly around the part having the compress laid on it. Leave it on for six to ten hours, remove, rinse the skin and dry thoroughly.

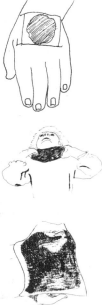

If an underpad is not available, the flax seed mixture can be spread on paper toweling of the appropriate size about 1/4 inch deep, covered with another layer of toweling and the compress placed on the affected part. A square of plastic must then be placed over the compress, with at least one inch edge overlap to prevent evaporation and leakage. Cover the entire compress with an old towel to catch leaks, and to hold in place. A binder or roller bandage may also be used to hold a charcoal compress in place, pinning or taping securely.

To make a charcoal compress for a bee sting, spider bite or other venomous bites, dissolve in water a spoonful or more of charcoal powder (enough to make sufficient paste to cover the area to be treated), or crush several tablets in plain water. Spread the paste on a folded piece of paper toweling large enough to cover the area to be treated and mold the compress to the area. The toweling should be thoroughly moistened with the paste. Cover the compress with a piece of plastic cut from a bread bag or other plastic bag, large enough to overlap the compress on all sides

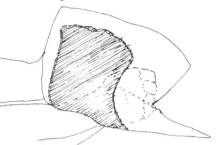

by at least one inch. A snug-fitting garment such as knitted cap can be used over a charcoal compress to hold it on the eye or over the sinuses or ear. A snug-fitting sweatshirt can hold a charcoal compress against the chest.

Hops from a health food store or smartweed (a common weed growing in most gardens) may be used to make a compress in the same way as the plain charcoal compress already described, the fresh or dried leaves being added to the paste by blending with a little water in a blender or crushing and adding directly to the paste. To convert this compress to a stupe, which may give a greater reaction, simply cover the compress which has been insulated by the plastic, with a fomentation or electric heating pad, and leave in place for about 20 minutes or more. Remove the fomentation or heating pad, dry off any excess moisture from around the compress, and cover well with a snug-fitting garment for the night, leaving the compress in place for the rest of the night.

CAUTION:

Care should be used in applying charcoal poultices to freshly broken skin. A tattooing effect is possible if a lesion extends into the dermis. For such wounds it is wiser to use comfrey poultices, avoiding the possibility of gaining an unwanted tattoo. There is little need to use a compress of any kind on a fresh wound, as charcoal is used for infection, inflammation, and swelling.

CHAPTER 4

IPECAC VERSUS CHARCOAL IN THE TREATMENT OF PEDIATRIC POISONINGS OR DRUG OVERDOSES

AVAILABILITY IN EUROPE

France and Belgium are far ahead of the United States in the use of activated charcoal as a first-line treatment for overdoses in the home and in the hospital. In these countries, activated charcoal is widely available in homes and pharmacies and is as accepted by parents for reserve in cases of accidental poisoning as Ipecac to induce vomiting is in this country. Parents have powdered charcoal in their medicine cabinets, but they have never heard 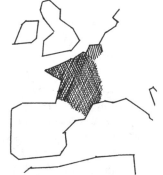 of Syrup of Ipecac. American pediatricians simply do not know to recommend charcoal for home use, despite the numerous reports of use for overdosage and poisonings in the American medical literature.

Considering the fact that Ipecac is itself a narcotic and is indeed not without hazard, plus the fact that Ipecac is not effective in causing vomiting in many children, nor does it work instantly as does charcoal, we present the superiority of charcoal over Ipecac in the following ways: 1) entirely safe; 2) has a much wider range of application than Ipecac; 3) is much cheaper than Ipecac; 4) has an indefinite shelf life; 5) works instantly on contact reducing the amount of the poison absorbed into the blood from the stomach. With Ipecac, there is a delay of up to 30 minutes before vomiting begins; and 6) Ipecac can be expected to get rid of only 25-35% of the poison, whereas charcoal eliminates 50-75%. If combined with vomiting induced by finger stimulation of the gag reflex, the proportion of elimination of poison should be increased another 10% or more.

There have been reports for many years that charcoal decreases absorption of many drugs. New evidence shows that charcoal actually doubles the elimination of overdoses of methylxanthines (caffeine, theobromine and theophyllin found in coffee, tea, colas and chocolate) and barbiturates over standard methods of treating toxins. Curtis and his co-workers showed that when comparing charcoal with Ipecac, charcoal comes out far ahead as being more effective. Curtis designed a program to test the efficacy of Ipecac alone versus activated charcoal plus a cathartic,versus the three together in the treatment of a simulated aspirin overdose. Seventy percent of the ingested aspirin dose turned up in the urine of patients following a standard Ipecac routine, indicating that it was absorbed into the body and passed through the kidneys. Only 56% of the dose was found in patients receiving activated charcoal. This presents impressive evidence for the greater effectiveness of activated charcoal in treating the overdose patient. Add to this its safety, long shelf life, low cost and ready availlity and its superiority as an antidote is clear.

Charcoal reaches its maximum rate of adsorption extremely rapidly; within one minute. In thick or viscid fluids such as the intestinal or stomach juices, adsorption might be delayed somewhat in actually touching the poison, but can still be expected to work very rapidly.

Like Syrup of Ipecac, Apomorphine brings up only about 30% of the poison in the stomach, meaning that they are inefficient in preventing poisoning by inducing vomiting, as 70% of the poison remains in the stomach.

ACTION AND CONTRAINDICATIONS
OF SYRUP OF IPECAC

Ipecac comes from Cartagena root, a Brazilian plant containing a number of poisonous alkaloids including emetine, cephaeline, emetamine and ipecamine. The plant also contains ipecacuantric acid and certain resins. The syrup has a clear amber color.

The reason Syrup of Ipecac acts to induce vomiting immediately after its administration is probably due to the highly irritating effect on the stomach by the major Ipecac alkaloids, emetine and cephaeline. After 20-30 minutes, vomiting is the result of absorption of these poisonous alkaloids with vomiting a result of stimulation of the central nervous system. About 93% of children will vomit within 30 minutes following one tablespoonful and two tablespoonsful for adolescents. The average time before vomiting is 20 minutes with a range between 14 and 30 minutes. During this time, the poison is being absorbed into the blood. If the person has lost the gag reflex or is having convulsions, or has taken strychnine, corrosives such as alkalis (lye) and strong acids, petroleum products (hydrocarbons) such as lighter fluid, kerosene or gasoline, fuel oil, paint thinner, or cleaning fluid, or any caustic substance, Ipecac should definitely not be given, as vomiting is contraindicated. While charcoal may not neutralize a great deal of these substances, it will do no harm and could do some good.

The emetine in Ipecac has cardiotoxic properties, that is, it will intoxicate the heart muscle, adding its own toxicity to the overall poisoned condition of the patient. With Ipecac alone, there may be continued nausea and vomiting beyond that expected, and also profuse diarrhea with cramping, fast heart rate with irregularities in the electrocardiogram (long PR interval, QRS changes, T-wave inversion), low blood pressure, muscle weakness, trembling and seizures. These effects may occur after a single large dose or repeated small doses of Ipecac. One person took Syrup of Ipecac daily for a two-month period to lose weight, developed heart rhythm irregularities and died.

Emetine has been reported to cause death from myocarditis. A torn place in the esophagus has also been reported, due to intensely forceful vomiting with Ipecac. With Ipecac, vomiting can be expected two or three times within an hour. If charcoal is given before Ipecac, the charcoal adsorbs the Ipecac, since Ipecac is itself poisonous. If the person fails to vomit with Ipecac, the *Physicians' Desk Reference* recommends that the dosage be recovered by washing the stomach, another potential complication with the use of Ipecac.

Lavage, or washing of the stomach, is another method for treating poisoning, but the use of charcoal is far more effective and easy. Charcoal is a home remedy whereas washing the stomach is a skilled technique, itself not without possibility of complication, such as perforation of the esophagus or stomach. Washing the stomach requires a trip to the emergency room and assembling a crew before the work can be done, often causing a delay of 30-90 minutes while the toxic material is being taken up. After the passage of the tube for stomach washing, the person has a sore throat for a day or two.

Charcoal is non-toxic, maintains its potency indefinitely in a closed container, and can be conveniently and safely administered in the home. There are no conditions that would be made worse by the primary use of charcoal. Even if it did no good, it will not harm. Activated charcoal is very well tolerated, even in amounts up to 100 grams (about one and three quarters cups of pulverized dry powder!).

There is no known contraindication to its use in acute poisonings. It is immediately effective and can be safely used by non- professionals. Charcoal is the most valuable single agent currently available for treating poisons. Babies and children accept 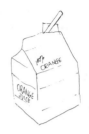 slurries made of water and powdered activated charcoal quite well. Serve in an orange juice carton, or opaque container with a straw.

Charcoal adsorbs well at body temperature, even better than at high temperatures. Heating to 350° in the oven can cause substances that have been adsorbed to be released. Charcoal can be reused once or twice by washing, settling, pouring off the fluid, and drying in the oven at a high temperature (350°).

Substances can be adsorbed by charcoal better from a water solution than from an organic solvent, such as alcohol, acetone, gasoline, etc. Nutrient salts such as sodium chloride and potassium nitrate are not readily adsorbed by activated charcoal. Iodine and mercuric chloride are well adsorbed. Simple acids and bases are easily adsorbed. Caustic materials are probably not readily adsorbed; therefore, when caustic agents such as lye have been swallowed, the offending agent may be poorly adsorbed unless large quantities of charcoal are used. While charcoal does no harm, it may not do much good with strong alkalis or strong acids, and more definitive treatment should be sought, such as drinking vinegar solution for alkalis and baking soda solutions for acids. The same may be true of the alcohols--methanol and ethanol (rubbing alcohol and beverage alcohol). There is experimental evidence in rats that charcoal is not effective in alcohol intoxication [4], although in humans, some have felt it has been effective in preventing intoxication.

In the past, some have wondered about the effect of acids or alkalis in the gastrointestinal tract on charcoal and its adsorbed materials, questioning whether poisons might become dislodged from the charcoal farther down and still wind up absorbed into the blood. It has been found that charcoal forms a stable complex with toxic materials, and washing with blood plasma or gastric juice fails to bring forth the toxic material from the charcoal. It has been bound so firmly that it will not be removed by ordinary means.[5]

SCORCHED FOOD NOT CHARCOAL

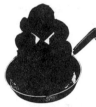

Charred food made in the kitchen from such items as burned bread or scorched food is definitely not charcoal. Scorched food has been found to be cancer-producing and is not recommended. Wood charcoal does not retain the harmful chemicals sometimes found in burned fats and protein (as these burn off), nor does it have mineral residues found in bone charcoal or scorched food.

MILK ACTS AS AN ANTIEMETIC

Sometimes advice is given to administer milk to children who have taken a drug or poison. Milk delays vomiting and the advice to give it is usually inappropriate.

SUBSTANCES ADSORBED BY CHARCOAL [6]

Acetaminophen	Mercuric chloride
Acetylcystine	(Mucomyst)Meprobamate
Aconite	Mercuric chloride
Aconitine	Methylene blue

Alcohol	Methyl salicylate
Amphetamine	Morphine
Antimony	Mucomyst
Antipyrine	Muscarin
Arsenic	Narcotics
Aspirin	Neguvon
Atropine	Nicotine
Barbital	Nortriptyline
Barbiturates	Opium
Cantharides	Oxylates
Camphor	Parathion
Carbon dioxide	Penicillin
Chlordane	Pentobarbital
Chloroquine	Pesticides
Chlorpheniramine	Phenobarbital
Chlorpromazine	Phenol
Cocaine	Phenolphthalein
Colchicine	Phenylpropanolamine
Cyanide	Phosphorus
Delphinium	Potassium cyanide
Delphinine	Potassium permanganate

2,4-Dichlorophenoxyacetic acid

	Primaquine
Digitalis	Propantheline
Diphenylhydantoin	Propoxyphene
Diphenoxylates	Quinacrine
Elaterin	Quinidine
Ergotamine	Quinine
Ethchlorvynol	Radioactive substances
Gasoline	Salicylamide
Glutethimide	Salicylates
Hemlock	Secobarbital
Hexachlorophene	Selenium
Imipramine	

Silver and some antimony salts

Iodine	Stramonium
Ipecac	Strychnine
Isoniazid	Sulfonamides
Kerosene	Tin

Lead acetate (to a limited extent)

Malathion	Titanium
Mefenamic acid	Veratrine

ASPIRIN OVERDOSE

Aspirin is the most commonly seen drug overdose, considering all ages, and charcoal quite effectively adsorbs aspirin. Symptoms of aspirin overdose include nausea and vomiting, rapid breathing, disorientation,

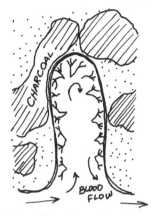

Microvillus of small intestine with location of charcoal in relation to blood shown.

and stomachache. With severe overdoses, coma and convulsions will be seen. The patient should be given 1-5 tablespoons of charcoal in water, and then large quantities of water (one 8 ounce glass every 10 minutes for the first hour, each with 1 teaspoon of charcoal, and thereafter, 1 glass per hour for 6 hours, then 1 glass every 2 hours for 12 more hours, each with charcoal) to protect the kidneys and to encourage elimination of aspirin. As soon as the overdose is recognized, charcoal should be administered, even if it is many hours after aspirin has been taken, as in the intestine charcoal performs a sort of dialysis, removing from the blood that circulates through the intestine many drugs that have long since passed through the stomach and gotten into the bloodstream.

Twelve adult volunteers were given 24 aspirin tablets. Three persons were used as controls, three were given two tablespoons of Syrup of Ipecac, repeated once if vomiting did not occur; three were given three teaspoons of magnesium sulfate (Epsom salts, a cathartic causing diarrhea) plus 60 grams of activated charcoal (about 1/2 cup of charcoal powder), and three patients were given both charcoal and Ipecac. Some aspirin turned up in the urine, indicating that certain portions of it were absorbed into the blood in all patients. With the aspirin alone, an average of 96% appeared in the urine.

With Ipecac alone, 70.3% appeared in the urine. With activated charcoal and magnesium sulfate, 56.4% appeared in the urine, and with all three, Ipecac, magnesium sulfate and activated charcoal, 72.4% appeared in the urine.

Activated charcoal and magnesium sulfate significantly reduced the absorption of aspirin. Ipecac alone or in combination with the other two failed to be as effective.[7] We believe charcoal alone would have been more effective than in combination with magnesium sulfate, as the salts slightly interfere with the action of charcoal.

DIAZEPAM (VALIUM) OVERDOSE

Diazepam is the second commonest overdose drug. There is no drug antidote and diazepam is not dialyzable with the artificial kidney. It is readily adsorbed by charcoal, and is the treatment of choice for diazepam overdoses.

TYLENOL POISONING

Acetaminophen (Tylenol) overdose is also common. It injures the liver and should be treated with both charcoal (1-5 tablespoons in water initially) and large doses of water (one glass every 10 minutes for the first hour, each glass with one teaspoon of activated charcoal powder) to dilute the effects on the liver. Charcoal also binds Mucomyst (acetylcysteine), the usual antidote for acetaminophen. Charcoal is as effective an antidote in Tylenol intoxication as is Mucomyst, and has no potential ill effects. It seems to us that since charcoal is less expensive, more readily available, has no serious side effects, and should be in every home medicine cabinet, that the treatment of choice should be listed as charcoal, not as acetylcysteine. This drug has many potential adverse reactions including sore mouth, nausea and vomiting, fever, runny nose, drowsiness, clamminess, chest tightness, and trouble breathing.

Alarming elevations in SGOT (a liver enzyme) often follow ingestion of acetaminophen (Tylenol), but a sizeable percentage of these patients recover. The dosage of charcoal should be repeated every two hours in the first six hours, along with 8 ounces of water each hour for an adult, and correspondingly less for a child. During the rest of the first 24 hours, give no food, but repeat the charcoal dosage and water every four hours to remove Tylenol from the blood through intestinal microdialysis. (**See Chapter Nine**).

TRICYCLIC ANTIDEPRESSANTS (TRIAVIL, ATIVAN, ETC.)

Tricyclic antidepressants are a cause of significant mortality in all ages, and is the number one cause of death by poisoning of children under age 10 in Alabama. They may be more severely intoxicating than their relative lack of symptoms may indicate. These patients may get high blood pressure and excitation, and with a high overdose, may get a fall in blood pressure, cardiac arrhythmias, coma, seizures, and finally death. Repeated charcoal treatments should be given to bind any active metabolites, either before absorption from the intestinal tract, or by being dialyzed from the bloodstream through the microdialysis system of the small bowel as described in **Chapter Nine**. Large quantities of fluid should be given to combat the fall in blood pressure. Tricyclic antidepressants are not dialyzable by the artificial kidney.[8]

CHAPTER 5

THE POISONED CHILD

Nothing strikes terror in the hearts of parents more than the chilling thought of their child taking something poisonous internally. I well remember the annual office-staff picnic in our back yard when my son was two and a half. All had been planned very carefully. The summer day had been characteristically hot prompting us to water down the lawn, concrete walks and patio very carefully, hoping later to benefit from the coolness the water carried into cracks, crevices and soil.

To further add to our comfort, I had purchased some brilliant purple fly tablets, the kind that makes flies lie on their backs with their legs poking uselessly up in the air. These were very carefully placed as far as my fingers could push them in the lattice brick work near the picnic table. That chore done, I very happily went about my business of making punch, getting hors d'oeuvres ready and supervising the kitchen. Soon the first of the guests began to arrive.

My husband and children seemed very happy to greet the office personnel, most of whom they knew by name. I was in and out of the house, preoccupied with my duties as hostess so only casually noticed traces of grape-colored material around my son's mouth. These I dismissed as remnants of some of the powdered material from an envelope he had been licking during the punchmaking. As I returned to the yard with a plate of pretzels, one of our guests, trying not to alarm me quietly said, "I believe your son has been eating fly tablets." In horror I looked at the grape-colored material around his mouth and recognized the deep purple of the fly tablets.

I took him in my arms to our large basement sink and held him against my left hip low on his own hips, tipping

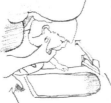

him over in a manner to force him to support his weight on the edge of the sink with his own two hands. I put my right hand as far back into his mouth as I could, and played a little tune on his tonsils and back of his throat. Fairly soon, he rewarded me by bringing up some punch, a good bit of gastric juice and four purple tablets. I had placed 12, so I continued to play my tune around his tonsils. Another reward of four more tablets. Another tune, and two more tablets. No amount of additional tune playing produced the last two so I assumed I had gotten back all he swallowed. I hurriedly went to the back yard and checked the places I could remember "hiding" the tablets and found the two missing ones.

After washing my son's face and changing his shirt, he was as good as new although we watched him very carefully for evidence of cholinesterase inhibitor toxicity for the next hour. From this time forth we began keeping charcoal in the medicine cabinet. Fortunately, we never had a similar cause for alarm, but the charcoal has been a good standby many a time through the years for indigestion, intestinal flatulence, nausea and vomiting, diarrhea, bee stings, toothache, earache, sore throats, headaches, and a hundred other ills.

For children under age five, medicines represent 40%

of the accidental poisonings. Cleaners and polishers 14.3%, plants 12.8%, cosmetics 10%, pesticides 5.5%, paints and solvents 4%, petroleum products 2.8% and gases and fumes 0.2%. Other or unknown products account for 10.4%

DIAGNOSIS OF POISONING

Prompt initial management of a case of poisoning is crucial. Children just don't "suddenly" become ill, and if they do, poisoning must always be suspected. **A child becoming lethargic, pale, weak, short of breath, or appears to be going unconscious is exhibiting danger signs. Symptoms such as confusion, seizure, inability to walk normally, blue lips or fingernails, rapid breathing, fast heart rate, burns in the mouth or throat, vomiting, or severe abdominal pain are also red flags.**

Check to see if the child has another cause for sickness such as a fever, sore throat, earache or other symptoms of infectious disease, and if anyone else in the family is ill. Could the child have fallen or had an accident, a blow to the head or an epileptic seizure? Is the child bruised or bleeding? Has the child or family recently gone through an unusual emotional stress such as attempted suicide, death of a family member, divorce, etc? An older child may have attempted suicide.

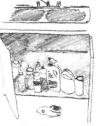

After considering these potential causes of sudden illness or injury, check to see if the child has been exploring under the kitchen sink or in the bathroom. Are any medicine bottles open or anything out of place in the house or garage? Determine if anyone in the household is taking medications--pain killers, tranquilizers, antidepressants, Lomotil, medication for bedwetting, iron tablets in pregnancy. Could the child have been exposed to alcohol or recreational drugs? Were unfinished alcoholic drinks left out in the child's vicinity? Check other symptoms of intoxication such as coughing, vomiting, diarrhea or headache. Does the child take insulin or any other kind of medication such as for heart or lung disease?

If it is known that a child took a certain medication, try to determine the maximum quantity the child could have taken, and exactly when the child would have swallowed it. How many tablets were in the bottle and how many are there now? How much is left of a container of liquid and how much was there in the beginning? When was the child last seen before being left unattended?

Symptoms are slow to appear sometimes if only a small amount of the poison has been swallowed. If a child has swallowed a small amount of kerosene and hasn't started to cough, choke or gag within 20-30 minutes, it is unlikely that there will be any respiratory problems.

After reading the preceeding few paragraphs, you may be wondering how you could carry out such an extensive investigation while little Johnny was sitting there holding his stomach and crying. Perhaps now would be the right time to repeat the oft quoted maxim, "An ounce of prevention is worth a pound of cure." Later in this chapter we talk about poison-proofing your home which is a vital and ongoing project. But in the case the worst ever happens, a calm head must prevail. Conducting the investigation with a prayer on the lips will sharpen your awareness and control your reason. It will also make any treatment you use far more effective.

HOW TO ADMINISTER CHARCOAL

The first aid treatment of choice is that of giving powdered charcoal stirred into a little water. Liquid or paste preparations available. It is quite likely that this will be the only treatment the child will need. On an empty stomach, the quantity of charcoal should be twice as much as the poison swallowed. Speed is highly desirable. Use two heaping tablespoons of the powder or 24 tablets broken up and crushed if you have no way to determine the quantity of the poison. Double this dosage if the child has eaten within two hours. Using up to eight to ten times the quantity of charcoal as the estimated weight of the poison is recommended by some if food is still in the stomach from the last meal (less than 3 hours). If the charcoal can be swallowed before the child becomes lethargic or in danger of being unable to swallow, much is gained. Don't use a large amount of water to stir the charcoal into, put a straw into it and suck it way back on the tongue and swallow quickly. A small child will struggle vigorously and will need to be held down. A spoon or ideally a 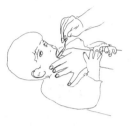 small bulb syringe can be used to transfer a small amount of the charcoal solution into the mouth. The child should be held in a position making swallowing the only option, preferably on the back. Then another small amount put into the mouth until the charcoal is all gone. (**Caution: Do not put anything in a child's mouth if sleepy, fainting or otherwise unable to swallow. In such cases, prompt professional attention is vital.**) The charcoal can be repeated as often as needed. Give plenty of water subsequently to insure easier passage of the charcoal.

A heaping tablespoonful of charcoal powder contains about five grams of charcoal. Mix it with a little water. One dose suffices for most ingestions. If the child vomits immediately after the initial dose, a second should be given promptly and given again and again until it is kept down. Give one heaping teaspoonful every hour thereafter for four hours and every four hours until a black stool is produced. To continue the dose every four hours until symptoms of intoxication are gone is quite appropriate if the substance swallowed is a cyclic antidepressant, barbiturate, theophylline, or salicylate, as

SYMPTOMS A CHILD MAY SHOW

ANTICHOLINERGIC DRUGS
(Atropine, Probanthine, Belladonnna, Fly Tablets and Spray)
dry mouth
facial flushing and no sweating
dilated pupils
fast heart rate

ASPIRIN
fast breathing
vomiting

DIGITALIS OR OTHER CARDIAC MEDICATION
vomiting
heart irregularity

OPIOIDS SUCH AS MORPHINE, DEMEROL AND OTHER ALKALOIDS
pinpoint pupils
shallow respirations
low blood pressure
skin cool to the touch
obtundation (dulling of mind)

CAUSTICS
(drain and toilet bowl cleaners, electric dishwasher detergents, phenol, Lysol)

pain and burning and swelling of the lips and mouth
hoarseness, difficulty and pain on swallowing
mouth filled with saliva
nose running
shallow breathing
weak, rapid pulse

PETROLEUM DISTILLATES
(gasoline, kerosene, lighter fluid, lacquer thinner, etc.)
coughing
choking
gagging
vomiting
hoarseness

these drugs and many others can be recycled through the intestinal tract after having been absorbed into the bloodstream, and taken up by charcoal during their trip through the bowel.

For further information on dosages see the end of this chapter.

SENSE OF SMELL IN IDENTIFYING UNKNOWN POISONS

POISON	*ODOR*
Cyanide	Bitter almonds
Alcohol or isopropyl alcohol	Fruit-like odor
Organophosphates	Garlic odor
Pyriminil (rat poison)	Peanuts
Nicotine	Stale tobacco
Urinary turpentine	Violets
Methylsalicylate	Wintergreen
Ethchlorvinol (Placidyl)	Pungent or aromatic odor

POISON-PROOF THE HOME

1. Move toxic substances from low shelves to high ones and make use of safety caps, latches and locks.

2. Don't leave cleaning agents or alcoholic drinks accessible and unattended.

3. Remove any toxic plants from your yard or home.

4. Store toxic substances only in their original containers.

5. Don't describe pills as candy to a child.

6. Throw away unused portions of medicines.

7. Be a responsible role-model and don't take medicines, alcoholic drinks, vitamins or herbal preparations in front of your child or he may try to imitate you.

8. Always keep activated charcoal in the house.

9. Keep the telephone number of your nearest regional poison control center and call that number first, instead of

your physician or the local poison control center. Valuable time may be lost, as persons in emergency rooms, physicians' offices, and even the local poison control center may not be as skilled in handling your particular child's problem as the regional poison control center.

CHARCOAL DOSAGE SCHEDULE*

Estimated total amount of poison or medicine taken	Charcoal powder to be used if person has not eaten in last 2 hours	Charcoal powder to be used if person has eaten in last 2 hours.
1 teaspoon, 1-2 tablets, 1-2 capsules	1-2 tablespoons of activated powder stirred in a little water. Rinse glass and drink rinsings. Follow by 2 glasses of water.	4-10 tablespoons activated powder stirred in a little water. Drink, rinse glass and drink rinsings. Follow by 2 glasses of water.
1 tablespoon, 3-5 tablets, 2-5 capsules	3-4 tablespoons of activated powder administered same as above.	6-15 tablespoons of activated powder administered same as above.
Unknown	1-5 tablespoons activated powder administered same as above.	5-15 tablespoons of activated powder administered same as above.

*Repeat all dosages in 30 minutes or if the symptoms begin to worsen. See text for rationale for treatment schedule.

CHAPTER 6

OVERDOSES AND TOXIC ACCIDENTS

MUSHROOM POISONING

Although mushrooms are consumed by the ton every day simmered in soups, sizzling on top of pizza, and sliced in light brown mounds in the "better" salad bars, there are probably few situations which can cause a sense of fear and distress more than that of going out in the back yard and picking your own "edible" fungus. The very thought of eating a poisonous mushroom is anathema, and for good reason.

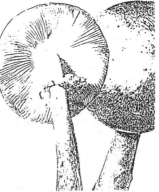

For the Amanita phalloides (the death cap) mushroom, treatment for ingestion has remained disappointing to medical science, not to mention those who accidently eat them. A wide variety of "cures" have been tried with sporadic success, among which have been prednisone, thioctic acid, vitamin C, penicillin, Cytochrome-C and hemodialysis alone or in combination with some of the above listed. But it has become common, if not readily accepted knowledge, that charcoal fixes or neutralizes the poison.

In one report, seven people were involved who had

eaten more than three mushrooms (three are generally considered a lethal dose), and did not seek treatment until 16 hours later. One of the four women was treated in a separate hospital from the other patients by an exchange transfusion and peritoneal dialysis. She went into hepatic coma for eight days and remained in the hospital for three months before she had recovered sufficiently to be sent home. Her husband, who had eaten the same quantity, was treated by hemoperfusion (filtering of the blood) using charcoal. He left the hospital after six days and was quite well. Four others left after three days. Since charcoal binds the toxic substance (alpha-amanitine) from water and protein solutions in artificial environments, it can be assumed it also does so inside the body as this case seems to indicate. The seven cases treated 16 hours after they had eaten the mushrooms indicate that charcoal can effectively remove the toxins from the blood even 24 hours after eating Amanita phalloides.[9]

Charcoal administration in the treatment of poisonings is increasing throughout the world. It is well recognized that charcoal has the ability to adsorb many toxins, and that drugs in the "enterohepatic circulation" (intestinal-liver circulation) can also be significantly cleared from the blood stream. Therefore repeated doses of charcoal, even many days after the ingestion of substances that remain in the blood a long time, is still a good treatment.

The administration of charcoal is indicated as the treatment of choice in almost all serious oral overdoses. Even in those cases where it is not an excellent remedy, it may still be the best available treatment, such as in alcohols, caustic agents, heavy metals (iron, mercury, lead, and so forth), and aliphatic hydrocarbons (gasoline, naphtha, kerosene, lighter fluid, etc.). One cannot go wrong by using charcoal in any intoxication. Even if it will do little good, it certainly will do no harm. In two instances where a drug antidote may be adsorbed to the charcoal, the charcoal is as effective as the traditional antidote, and nothing is lost by giving the charcoal.

These two instances are Syrup of Ipecac to induce vomiting and the use of Mucomyst for acetaminophen (Tylenol) overdose. Mucomyst and acetaminophen are both effectively adsorbed to charcoal, and the patient may be completely treated provided sufficient charcoal is administered to take care of all the toxic substances - Ipecac or Mucomyst - as well as acetaminophen, for which the first two drugs may have been given as antidotes.

America is certainly on the brink of a major change in routine for the overdose patient. The extensive experience with charcoal in Europe has prompted this trend as American doctors are beginning to recommend activated charcoal as a first line treatment for most acute poisonings. The editorial board for Poisindex, the most widely used primary poison information system, decided to make this change in most of the 291 treatment protocols, as of January 1985.[10]

Herbicides applied liberally or having an inordinately long residual effect, may be efficiently counteracted by a charcoal spray. Simply take the garden sprayer, fill it with a charcoal suspension, and spray it to your heart's content.

It has been used to remove toxins from the blood in kidney and hepatic diseases, taking the charcoal internally or applying it as a compress or both, and for use in an exchange column to perfuse blood.

Charcoal effectively inhibits theophylline absorption into the blood. In one study, an average of only 40% of the administered dose was absorbed into the bloodstream in the presence of activated charcoal, even if charcoal was administered 30 minutes after taking the test dose of theophylline.[11] In another study, theophylline in the serum was reduced to about one-third by taking activated charcoal.[12] That study illustrates the capabilities of charcoal in removing from the blood toxic substances by the method of micro-dialysis described in chapter nine.

Therefore, always bear in mind the speed with which the charcoal is administered will determine to a certain degree the success in combating poisons, but that the dosage should be repeated occasionally during the first day or two after poisoning to remove any breakdown products from the intestinal tract, or poison that may be recycled through the blood vessels of the intestine.

CHAPTER 7

IMPORTANT TREATMENTS
WITH CHARCOAL

DIARRHEA

Perhaps one of the most effective uses for charcoal is in cases of diarrhea. It has been used by soldiers in time of war for both the prevention and treatment of diarrhea.[13] About the same time the French reported benefits from charcoal in military campaigns, the German literature also carried similar reports.[14] Soldiers carried the custom of using charcoal back home to their families, and the custom has since spread all over Europe.

In diarrhea caused by cholera, two heaping teaspoons of powdered charcoal should be given four times daily as well as with each loose stool. All the fluid one can take by mouth should also be supplemented with one to two and a half liters of normal saline intravenously or per rectum or subcutaneous push-in. Since severe dehydration characterizes cholera, it must be fought from the beginning of treatment. When patients die, it is usually not of toxicity but of dehydration.[15] Treat dehydration with vegetable broth to which $^1/_2$ to 1 teaspoon of salt has been added per pint. Measure the quantity of fluid lost in stools and urine and replace that much, plus the usual 8 glasses (8 ounces each) daily with some extra if there is a fever with sweating. With great care and diligence, these patients can be saved.

One group of young girls and their leader went for a

39

four day camping trip in the woods. They built a campfire, ate the picnic lunch they had brought with them, and everyone went to bed. During the night several of the girls began to have diarrhea. By morning the leader and all of the girls felt bad and most of them had diarrhea. By nightfall they were all suffering from the diarrhea. The camp counselor wondered what she should do - should she take the entire group home, should they tough it out, should she call a doctor? She had heard charcoal was good for diarrhea, and as she sat gazing into the fire she decided she would try making her own charcoal. She took several pieces of partly burned wood from the fire, rinsed the ash off, and chewed as much of the charred wood to a fine powder as possible. Within an hour she was feeling entirely well. She convinced four of the eight girls to chew some of the charred wood pieces. Each girl who tried it was well within an hour. Those who could not bring themselves to chew on the charred wood continued to be sick throughout the entire camping trip.

The dosage of charcoal for diarrhea is the full dose given repeatedly, one dose with each loose stool. Use one heaping tablespoon stirred into water for an adult and a correspondingly smaller dose for a child.

NAUSEA AND VOMITING

Another of the most effective treatments with charcoal is for nausea and vomiting. Give the full adult dose - one to two heaping tablespoonsful stirred in a little water, or approximately half that for a child-- each time a vomiting episode occurs. If the charcoal is vomited, more should be given again in full dosage immediately. Even if the charcoal has to be given again and again, it will prove well worth the effort. Always follow the dose with a full glass or two of water.

We have never seen a case of acute nausea and vomiting in which treatment was begun early that continued past three doses of charcoal kept down. We believe it to be the most effective treatment available for nausea and vomiting and should always be used as the primary treatment of choice. Often very uncomfortable patients will feel well in seconds after swallowing the charcoal slurry made from charcoal powder stirred in water.

EFFECT OF CHARCOAL ON CANCER-PRODUCING COMPOUNDS

A study of carbon black (bone charcoal) revealed that when applied by itself it will not cause tumors, whether fed, painted, or injected subcutaneously in olive oil suspension. It has not been known to produce a single benign or malignant tumor in 460 animal trials. It was shown that the carcinogenicity of p-dimethylaminoazobenzene (azo dye) was almost completely abolished by carbon black. Only one of seventy-two animals fed azo dye adsorbed onto carbon black developed a hepatoma. Usually almost 100% develop tumors called hepatomas.

Charcoal can adsorb other cancer-producing agents such as methylcholanthrine and benzpyrene. These are chemicals which, when applied to the skin, are capable of producing cancer. They can also be effectively adsorbed and inactivated by charcoal.[16] These prominent cancer producing agents are formed when beef steak is grilled because of scorching the fat.

Administration of carbon black-adsorbed cholanthrene and benzpyrene inhibited their carcinogenesis, making them not at all carcinogenic with charcoal. However, carcinogenicity in the two compounds was restored when olive oil or acetone were allowed to act for weeks or months on the charcoal-adsorbed substance before injecting.[17]

ANEMIA OF CANCER

In cancer patients who are anemic the administration of charcoal will sometimes cause a reversal of the anemia since anemia in cancer patients is caused by a toxicity from the cancer itself. To administer charcoal may remove the toxic substance which inhibits the bone marrow, thereby allowing the bone marrow greater freedom in performing its ordinary functions.

DIABETES MELLITUS

Charcoal has been used in the treatment of patients with diabetes mellitus. The adsorption of glucose by charcoal occurring in the bowel has resulted in some patients being able to take a decreased dosage of insulin or oral sugar-reducing agents. Charcoal has also caused a reduction of signs of blood vessel and nerve pathology, the most dreaded complications of diabetes. There has been also a normalizing of the activity of digestive organs. The triglycerides in some studies tended to decrease and the atherogenic index went down.[18] These are all salutary effects in diabetes, reducing some of the most troublesome symptoms and side effects.

OXYGEN APPLIED TO SKIN BY CHARCOAL

Charcoal adheres to oxygen, taking it along with it into all its treatment situations. If oxygen is intended to be added to any lesion, such as in diabetic gangrene, one way to deliver oxygen to the tissues directly could be through the application of a generously made charcoal compress. The presence of oxygen on charcoal was discovered in hemoperfusion for temporary artificial liver support.[19]

OTHER WELL KNOWN USES
OF CHARCOAL

Intestinal gas and intestinal disorders may also be treated with charcoal. The area in which charcoal is being most widely recognized and written up in many different kinds of medical and health publications is as an effective method of controlling intestinal gas. Although it is an old fashioned remedy as pointed out in **Chapter 2**, it works better than simethicone, the agent now commonly used for this purpose. Charcoal was once widely used, both here and in Europe for gas, but became displaced by the product having greater commercial attractiveness. Recently charcoal has again become widely used for this purpose.

It is also used in making medicines, coloring candy (jelly beans), and making licorice candy.

CHAPTER 8

DEODORIZING WITH CHARCOAL

HOUSEHOLD

That charcoal could be used in refrigerators and closets has only recently been widely realized. A good way to accomplish this deodorizing task is to place some powdered charcoal in a pint jar with a screw cap which has many holes punched in it, replace the cap and put the jar in a place unlikely to be tipped over. It can be placed in dresser drawers, closets, pet areas, or under the house where an odor has developed.

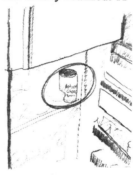

A friend of ours was visited by a friendly skunk who made a nest under her house. Her husband took measures to remove the skunk, but the skunk left abundant evidence of his having been in the area. Powdered charcoal was sprinkled over the area which brought deodorizing in a matter of minutes.

If a refrigerator must sit unused for some time, a pint jar with charcoal as previously described can be placed in it with the most excellent results of deodorizing.

(Always insure that an unused refrigerator or freezer cannot be turned into a death-trap for an exploring child by removing its latching devices or somehow locking it shut.)

Rancid odors in the kitchen may be effectively removed by charcoal in an open container. Charcoal has been used in cigarette filters but we would draw the line in declaring the use of tobacco safe because charcoal was introduced. Nothing but abstinence makes cigarettes safe.

In recent years charcoal has been used with skin ulcers, orthopedic casts, and internally to deodorize breath or bowel. Surgeons often put an ileostomy or colostomy patient on a small dose of charcoal two to four times a day (usually one half teaspoonful in a single dose is effective). The foul odors from bowel incontinence can be immediately corrected by activated charcoal enemas, or by giving charcoal by mouth. The foul odor of inoperable cancer of the cervix can be readily relieved by a douche using a solution of charcoal powder stirred into the douche water - two tablespoons of powdered activated charcoal in a quart of water (or a pint if preferred).[20]

SUBMARINES

Because charcoal is effective in combating odors in air and water, and because it is quite effective in removing carbon dioxide from air, it is used extensively in submarines, in fact, the submarine industry is entirely dependent on charcoal. Filters in gas masks to remove poison is also a common use of charcoal.

BAD BREATH

Willow charcoal, or any commercial charcoal, is quite effective against bad breath. Since 90 percent of bad breath arises in the mouth, to swish charcoal around in the mouth or to hold a charcoal tablet in the mouth will stop bad breath immediately.

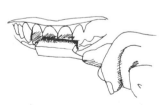

ORTHOPEDIC CASTS, WOUNDS, AND SKIN PROBLEMS

Charcoal has been used in open draining wounds bandaged in plaster cast immobilization. This kind of wound is a common problem for the orthopedic surgeon. The odor coming from a draining wound inside a cast makes frequent cast changes necessary. At Fort Benning, Georgia, Dr. Frank Haydon developed a technique to avoid such frequent changes. He took fifteen grams of activated charcoal (about three to four tablespoons) and mixed it with enough water to make a slurry. After the first layer of cast was applied, the charcoal slurry was then poured over the area of expected drainage. The remainder of the plaster was then applied over this wet charcoal. The cast appeared slightly gray but was accepted well by patients. The unacceptable odor of draining wounds was controlled for much longer periods of time with no adverse effect on wound or fracture.[21]

Lesions caused by Bacillus pyocyanase can be quite nicely deodorized by the use of charcoal. Healing is also improved, as the charcoal takes up bacteria. One good way to apply charcoal to a foul smelling ulcer is by putting some of the powder in a salt shaker with a few grains of rice. Shake the powdered charcoal on the wound with every bandage change. The foul odor is dissipated in one treatment.[22] Eczema has also been successfully treated using charcoal, especially where there is infection and odor.[23]

We had a patient who had a large, deep ulcer (12 inches in diameter) due to an x-ray burn on the back from an overdose of x-ray used for treating a skin cancer. The ulcer became infected and foul smelling. His entire house smelled of the ulcer, despite the most fastidious care. We started dressing the ulcer by sprinkling dry charcoal from a salt shaker on all the moist areas before applying gauze. Instantly the odor vanished from the ulcer and gradually left the house. Although the patient eventually succumbed to the radiation sickness, he and his whole family were grateful for the charcoal.

Charcoal cloth has been used in the management of discharging, infected, and malodorous wounds. In varicose leg ulcers and in infected surgical wounds, a single layer of charcoal cloth covered with a porous fabric sleeve dressing gave a noticeable reduction in wound odor in 95% of 39 patients. Wound cleansing was also noted in 80 %. There were no adverse reactions to the material. The dressings did not stick to the wounds and could be removed without difficulty. Charcoal cloth also adsorbs bacteria.[24]

CHAPTER 9

MICRODIALYSIS OF THE BLOOD BY CHARCOAL

Since charcoal can effectively take up a wide variety of poisons when mixed directly with it, we would

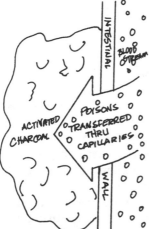

expect charcoal would work very effectively in the stomach to take up poisons and medicines. It is less evident, however, that charcoal could remove or extract poisons from the blood after the poisons have been taken up from the gastrointestinal tract, or even when they have been injected into the bloodstream.

Recent experiments have shown conclusively that activated charcoal not only takes up drugs in the stomach, small intestine, and colon, but can attract drugs from the blood back into the gastrointestinal tract where charcoal takes it up and inactivates it. This has been called "gastrointestinal dialysis".

Phenobarbital and Other Drugs

When charcoal was given by mouth on repeated occasions in patients who had taken intravenous phenobarbital or theophylline, the rate of elimination of these drugs was doubled and the half life of the drug markedly reduced! Since the kidney clearance and the liver metabolism were not affected by activated charcoal, the drugs already in the plasma must cross the blood vessel and intestinal membranes and be secreted into the intestine to be taken up by the charcoal in the intestine. We recommend that charcoal be given following overdoses from theophylline or phenobarbital every two to four hours until the patient is completely out of danger. The dosage suggested by authors of the above study was about one gram per kilogram, or about one half to one cup of charcoal powder stirred into sufficient water to make a slurry, and then sucked up through a straw.[25]

In normal volunteers who had taken an oral dose of phenobarbital, carbamazepine, or phenylbutazone, charcoal administered ten hours later was very effective. Blood studies showed that absorption into the bloodstream was essentially completed before charcoal was administered. There was a marked decrease in drug concentrations beginning shortly after charcoal was swallowed. The biologic half life of phenobarbital decreased on the average from 110 hours to 19.8 hours, that of carbamazepine from 32 to 17.6 hours, and that of phenylbutazone from 51.5 to 36.7 hours. Patients who were given activated charcoal by nasogastric tube for severe phenobarbital intoxication recovered consciousness much sooner than expected from their blood levels of phenobarbital. The half life became less than 24 hours rather than the usual half life of about 100 hours. The same thing has been done with Digitoxin through repeated oral doses of activated charcoal, exhibiting increased systemic elimination.[26]

Linden and his helpers reported on the use of charcoal for persons who had received phenobarbital as an overdose. When they received multiple doses of charcoal their phenobarbital half life was found to be 24 hours compared with 73 hours for their controls. We can say, therefore, that drugs are not only adsorbed by charcoal from the gastrointestinal tract, but can be attracted from the general circulation back into the gastrointestinal tract, there to be taken up by charcoal.[27] It is important in cases of poisoning to continue to give charcoal for several days after the patient seems to recover from the acute poisoning.

The microdialysis occurs from the capillary network of the villus to the charcoal granules in the intestine lumen.

Theophylline Intoxication:

Two patients had the heart signs of theophylline toxicity (atrial fibrillation in both cases) as well as gastrointestinal complaints and neurologic symptoms (agitation). About 30 grams (6 tablespoons) of oral charcoal were given every two to four hours for four doses. The signs and symptoms cleared promptly. By

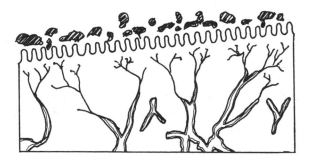

Microdialysis occurs from the capillary network of the villus to the charcoal granules.

many observations and experiments we can see that oral charcoal is quite effective in increasing the clearance and removal of theophylline from the blood. Therefore, inhaled intoxicants or injected substances can be expected to clear from the blood faster if charcoal is given by mouth on a continual basis until the blood is clear.[28]

51

CHAPTER 10

THE VETERINARY USE OF CHARCOAL

Early in our experience with using charcoal on humans, we wondered if animals might also be benefitted by its healing properties. We did not have long to wait, as one of our neighbor's pet cats had a fight with a neighboring cat and sustained wounds that became infected. We sprinkled charcoal from a salt shaker directly into the infected area and witnessed a marvelous transformation. In hours the wound crusted over, and in a day or two had a nice slough with pink skin underneath.

A lady veterinarian told us of a horse which injured his foot by kicking the corral fence. The wound was swollen, infected, and painful. We gave her some charcoal to sprinkle into the wound. She was very pleased with the prompt improvement where antibiotics had been fruitless.

The habu, a well-known venomous reptile on the island of Okinawa, is responsible for great disability and death there every year. It is so bad the government sponsors an annual drive to try to reduce the habu population before rice-harvesting time. Just before our visit there in the summer of 1982, a pet kid belonging to some friends of ours had been bitten by a large habu. When they found it, its head and neck were extremely swollen, and the little goat, bleating inconsolably, could not stand.

Rather than abandoning it to its fate, some young men set about to try saving it. They decided on a remedy which they had used often on humans for wasp stings, spider bites, and poison ivy, but had never used for snakebites.

They dug a deep hole in the ground and filled it with a mixture of water, clay, and charcoal. The kid was laid in, and the boys took turns holding its nose above water. Although it seemed to get stronger, the boys soon tired, and since nightfall was approaching, they left the animal to fend for itself. Next morning they went back, expecting to find him dead. To their amazement, the kid had climbed out of the hole, and was grazing quietly nearby, with most of the swelling gone. We can definitely say that charcoal and clay are useful for habu-bitten goats!

Charcoal has been administered quite successfully to sheep and cattle for lantana poisoning. Lantana is a plant which grows in pastures. Children and animals can become poisoned by this plant. The report of the successful administration of activated charcoal for the treatment of lantana poisoning of sheep and cattle was made in the <u>Journal</u> <u>of</u> <u>Applied</u> <u>Toxicology</u>.[29]

Another incident which took place in Missouri in 1985, involved a horse with a hopelessly infected eye.

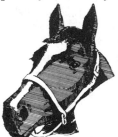

The horse was in a group of other horses being offered for sale, but because of its eye, seemed destined for destruction. One family, intending only to buy a small pony from the owner, agreed to purchase the injured one also for an additional $25. At least the saddle was worth that much, they reasoned. Little hope was given for the poor animal.

The family immediately went to work on the eye, which, when delivered, had become a sickening mass of oozing puss giving no evidence an eye was even present in the socket anymore. Twice daily, charcoal poultices sprinkled with golden seal were applied to the eye, held in place by a nylon stocking. Charcoal, flax seed and apples were also blended together and fed to the filly. Within weeks the eye had cleared up and she was as sound as the other horses. Less than a year later a beautiful, healthy foal was born to her. As of this writing she gives no indication she once had such a unsightly malady.

One more incident from the Ozarks took place under similar circumstances. A Rhode Island Red hen, which had been attacked by a neighbor's dog, was placed in a cardboard box apparently awaiting its inevitable end. Although no wounds were readily visible, it did not, or could not, rise when approached by strangers. The owners gladly gave the hapless bird to the first willing people happening along who just happened to be the owners of the previously mentioned horse. She really looked fine... from the top.

Upon arriving back at their own farm, they took "Hanna" out of the box to examine the cause of her reluctance to get up and scratch around like her ancestors had done for thousands of fowl generations. They were not prepared for what met their eyes. Hidden under a writhing mass of maggots lay the exposed labyrinth of her intestines. The smell was as foul as the sight, prompting a first reaction to just put her out of her misery. But she sat there so patient, so trusting, so...well, full of faith. It seemed a shame to exercise less faith than a chicken, so out came the charcoal.

Her bed was dusted heavily with the black powder and she was also fed liberal amounts of charcoal in her feed and water. Recovery, which included lots of time in the open air and sunshine, was rapid and soon she was queen of the yard, playing mother to the six Banties sharing her domain. Charcoal had once again preserved health in the barnyard.

CHAPTER 11

SUBSTANCES NOT
ADSORBED BY CHARCOAL

While there are no true contraindications for using activated charcoal, (even for Tylenol intoxication in which it also takes up the antidote - Mucomyst, quite well) there are some cases where charcoal would be ineffective. While no damage would be done by the use of charcoal, little good could be expected either, making it better to start with some other treatment, if available, from the beginning.

One such case is in iron intoxication. Children often find the enticing candy-coated iron tablets mother is taking for a subsequent pregnancy, and eat numerous pills. Iron is irritating to the gastrointestinal tract and can be fatal in children with overdosage. Since charcoal binds nutrients very poorly, iron is bound poorly by charcoal and the child is not helped significantly by the administration of charcoal. Putting the fingers down the throat of the child and massaging vigorously the tonsils and root of the tongue is the treatment of choice. When all possible 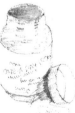 tablets have been recovered, give a child's size glass of water every 10 minutes for an hour, and one glass every hour for 6 hours, then one glass every 2 hours for 12 hours, each glass of water with one teaspoon of charcoal stirred in.

The ingestion of caustic substances, both strong acids

as well as strong alkali, should be treated by neutralizing the substance - vinegar water for alkalis such as lye, and baking soda water for acids such as hydrochloric. It will do no harm to give large quantities of charcoal in these poisonings, especially as a first aid measure, as charcoal does adsorb some acids and alkalis.

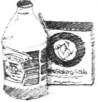

Charcoal would not interfere with examination of oral or esophageal burns as the burns would be highlighted, rather than obscured, by charcoal. Normal mucosa is not stained by charcoal in the slightest but rinses off promptly. Charcoal not only does not interfere with the healing process of caustic burns, but retards bacterial growth and inhibits infection.

Some alcohols are adsorbed by charcoal, but methanol and ethanol are not adsorbed. Methanol is sometimes used as rubbing alcohol, and ethanol is beverage alcohol.

Elemental metals such as iron and lithium, as well as some non-metals such as boron are poorly adsorbed onto charcoal. Some pesticides such as malathion, DDT, and carbonate are also poorly adsorbed. It has been said that

cyanide is not adsorbed onto charcoal, but that may be because cyanide is so quickly lethal there is no time to administer the charcoal.[31]

CHAPTER 12

DOES CHARCOAL INTERFERE WITH DIGESTION OR NUTRIENT ABSORPTION?

To test if charcoal interferes with the absorption of nutrients from the gastrointestinal tract into the bloodstream, a number of different kinds of observations can be made. A simple study can be done on persons having ostomies.

An ileostomy or colostomy patient is often given charcoal in small doses intermittently throughout the day to cut down on odors and gas. Although these patients are nutritionally compromised from their surgery, they do not seem to have any problem resulting from taking charcoal; in fact, many ostomy patients will take a small dose of charcoal daily for years, with no notable adverse effect. We do not believe there is significant interference with nutrient absorption from the intestinal tract by charcoal.

Persons with bad breath have taken small doses of charcoal throughout the day to combat bad breath of a metabolic source. Bad breath arising in the mouth can also be treated by a charcoal mouth wash as readily as by swallowing charcoal. Just as the ostomy cases, these patients also seem to tolerate charcoal on a long term basis quite well.

Charcoal added to the diet of sheep for six months did not cause a loss of nutrients when compared with sheep not receiving charcoal. Blood tests showed no significant difference between the two groups of animals and there were no visible signs of any nutritional deficiency. At autopsy no differences, either grossly or microscopically could be detected. A level of five percent of the total diet was given as charcoal. No effect could be detected on urinary levels of calcium, copper, iron, magnesium, inorganic phosphorus, potassium, sodium, zinc, creatinine, uric acid, urea, nitrogen, alkaline phosphatase, total protein, or urine pH. Although the animals inhaled some of the powdered charcoal there were no ill effects detectable in the microscopic sections of the lungs or other structures of the chest.[31]

Workers in charcoal manufacturing plants show no increase in incidence of respiratory symptoms, indicating that breathing the dust is quite innocuous.[32]

In the Journal of the American Medical Association for December 7, 1957, a small article appeared suggesting there were no known chronic deleterious effects from ingesting powdered charcoal in small amounts over long periods of time. A reference was cited that activated charcoal will remove many irritating substances - toxic amines, organic acids of decomposed foods, and even bacteria.[33]

Emery, in the Journal of the American Medical Association in 1937, suggested that activated charcoal might adsorb enzymes, vitamins, and minerals, but subsequent investigation has shown that if nutrients or normal body products are taken up at all, it is very poorly with wood charcoal.

Blood charcoal mixed with a diet of polished rice fed to rats and pigeons produced symptoms of malnutrition quicker and more severely than on white rice alone, but that was only when large amounts of charcoal were given. When one considers giving a half-teaspoonful two to four times daily for a chronic condition such as bad breath, it hardly seems worthwhile to mention an amount that small.

Three studies were conducted in France during the

mid-1940's on young rats. The first, reported in the French literature in 1945, was favorable toward charcoal. In it, two groups of rats were tested to determine if one group fed with an identical diet with another group could be made to have a deficiency disease by including charcoal. It was discovered the two groups were identical with or without charcoal.[34]

The other two seemed to indicate that charcoal interferes with certain nutrients. These are the only two studies that seem to indicate such a problem, but the complete methodology of the experiments was not included in the reports making significant findings far less meaningful. These two studies are outlined below.

One study reported in the French medical literature entitled "The Effect of Charcoal on the Utilization of Vitamins in a Balanced Diet" compared two groups of young rats, one given a complete mixed diet, and the second group given the same kind of diet mixed with animal or vegetable charcoal. The growth rate was retarded in all animals receiving charcoal. There was a marked lowering in the excretion of vitamin B-1 and riboflavin, but little effect on nicotinic acid and pantothenic acid. Even when extra doses of vitamin B-1 and riboflavin were given the amounts excreted were much lower in rats having the charcoal. Whether this effect was due to displacing food in the diet because of the mixing in of charcoal was not discussed in the translation we examined. So far as we know, this study has not been repeated since originally reported in 1948.[35] More recent studies show very poor adsorption of vitamins and minerals or other nutrients by charcoal.

The other was reported in 1945 in the French medical literature under the title, "Diets Containing Activated Charcoal and Early Development of Vitamin-A Deficiency". A group of twelve young rats receiving a diet deficient in vitamin-A survived about 100 days while a group receiving the same diet with two percent charcoal added survived only about 50 days. Again it was not discussed as to whether the charcoal displaced some portions of food from the diet, or if it actually took up vitamin-A or other nutrients. There have been no additional studies which would indicate a particular affinity by charcoal for vitamins A, B-1, or riboflavin.

CHAPTER 13

SUBSTANCES MIXED WITH CHARCOAL TO MAKE IT MORE PALATABLE OR EFFECTIVE

Since charcoal has a very black color it is not appealing to children, even though it is tasteless and odorless. The texture of grittiness in the mouth adds nothing to its acceptability.

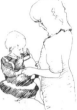

A very good way to make the suspension palatable is to pour it into a chocolate milk carton, add a couple of large straws and offer the mixture graciously to the patient. If a name such as "chalk-a-sorb" is given to the suspension, it will be even more acceptable, as it sounds somewhat like chocolate.

The mixing of a fructose solution with a super active charcoal resulted in twice as much aspirin being adsorbed in volunteers as compared with ordinary activated charcoal.[36]

Sometimes substances such as sorbitol are mixed with charcoal along with flavoring agents to try to make it more acceptable and easier to use in emergency departments. While the acceptability is better, the sorbitol interferes slightly with the effectiveness of charcoal. The mixing of powdered charcoal into plain water is actually only a minor problem. Charcoal powder has an indefinite shelf life, remaining effective for years, probably decades.

The "universal antidote," a combination of milk of magnesia, ordinary grocery tea, and charcoal has been used in emergency rooms around the country for over one hundred years. This antidote is decidedly inferior to plain charcoal, the tannic acid in the tea decreasing the effectiveness of charcoal, and the milk of magnesia interfering with the adsorption. Tannic acid as found in many herbs precipitates alkaloids, certain glycosides, and many metals. It reduces the usefulness of charcoal as an antidote. In most emergency rooms the universal antidote has been abandoned and charcoal alone is now being used.

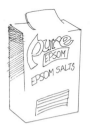

Magnesium sulfate, a standard saline cathartic marketed under the name "Epsom salts," has been used with charcoal to hasten the passage of charcoal with its adsorbed material through the gastrointestinal tract. A cathartic by itself will prevent some of the absorption of poisonous substances by the gastrointestinal tract. It has been felt that a cathartic would help to prevent retention of the charcoal in the intestinal tract. However, many poisons are themselves cathartic, and the addition of a cathartic such as epsom salts could be more distressing and physically taxing to the patient.

Because of the unpleasant taste of magnesium sulfate, the addition of this cathartic to charcoal reduces its palatability and acceptance by patients. Since charcoal does not allow the poisonous substances adsorbed to "desorb" along the intestinal tract, we feel that the cathartic is unnecessary and will actually add to the problems of administration of charcoal.

To the present time no good tests have been done to determine if epsom salts would interfere with the adsorptive qualities of charcoal.

SPECIFIC CONDITIONS TREATED

BEE STINGS, YELLOW JACKETS, Etc.

Externally, venomous bites can be readily treated with charcoal. Fire ants leave a sterile abscess from the venom which kills a tiny area of tissue. An ordinary band-aid, wet slightly, and rubbed with a charcoal tablet until entirely black and applied as a mini-poultice combats ant stings. The same treatment is effective for mosquito and chigger bites, and small areas of poison ivy.

The perfect treatment for bee stings is a charcoal compress. We believe that first aid is best administered in the form of charcoal to those that are intensely allergic to bee stings. We recommend that such individuals take a small quantity of charcoal with them when they go into areas where they might be stung. Mixing a bit of charcoal with water and smearing it over the bee sting area could be life saving.

For venomous bites or poison ivy, immediately wash the area well with soap and water, or flood with a solution of charcoal. After this brief preparation, the charcoal compress can be applied. Ven- 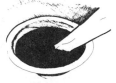 omous bites may be submerged in cool charcoal water for an hour and followed by a compress. Use 1/2 cup of charcoal to about 2-5 gallons of water.

CASE HISTORIES

A three-year old girl was playing in her yard. Seeing a hole in the ground, her curiosity was piqued and she stuck a stick into it. Out came a swarm of angry <u>yellow jackets</u>, which immediately attacked her. Hearing her screams, her mother came running to the rescue. By that time the little girl was covered with the vicious insects; we later counted over fifty stings on her from the collar bones up. The frantic mother began to beat them off, in the process getting fifteen or twenty stings herself. Hearing her call for help, several people came running. They immediately placed the girl in a tub of cool water and stirred several tablespoons of charcoal into it, covering everything except her nose and mouth, and keeping her there for about thirty minutes. After cleaning her up, she seemed perfectly comfortable, and soon was playing again. The mother, who had been too busy to care for her own stings, had marked swelling and pain that persisted for several days.

Mrs. T. had become extremely allergic to <u>bee stings</u>. With her last sting, she had nausea, weakness, faintness, 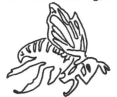 and some wheezing, which had necessitated treatment at an emergency room. Her physician had warned her that the next attack could be fatal, and urged her to undergo a series of desensitization shots. Unfortunately, before she could do so, she got another sting on her hand. Right away, the lady was pale, sweaty, weak, had a headache and nausea, and severe pain in her hand. She was beginning to wheeze.

We first rubbed the sting with a charcoal tablet wet with water as the very quickest way to apply the charcoal, and immediately mixed some activated charcoal and water, and more completely covered the sting. Within 2 or 3 minutes of the charcoal application, she began to relax and feel better. A larger poultice was prepared to replace the emergency one, and it was changed at 10 minute intervals for an hour. We gave her a tablespoon of charcoal by mouth in a glass of water. Then an interesting thing happened.

The patient felt perfectly well and took the poultice off believing herself to be entirely finished with the reaction. Within 10 minutes, she was weak, sweaty, faint, and beginning to wheeze. The poultice was immediately re-applied, again with clearing of symptoms. After wearing the poultice all night, she was well. Although this lady usually experienced massive swelling after bee stings, she had no trace of swelling to develop.

SNAKEBITES

We have not yet had first-hand experience in treating snakebites with charcoal, but physicians who have successfully used it find it a good 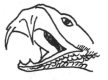 treatment. In isolated areas where antivenin is unavailable, and for snakebites for which there is no antivenin, we would immediately apply a very large charcoal compress covering almost an entire extremity, centering over the bite, using large quantities of activated charcoal wet with water and kept moist by covering with plastic. A new compress should be placed over the immediate vicinity of the snakebite every ten to fifteen minutes. Activated charcoal should also be taken by mouth, in the quantity of approximately two tablespoonsful every two hours for three doses, and one teaspoonful every four hours for the next 24 hours. Each dose should be followed by two glasses of water.

The sooner charcoal is applied, the more effective the treatment should be. Swelling and pain are evidences of envenomation in a snakebite. The swelling should be in evidence within ten minutes of being bitten or one should question whether there has been envenomation. We recommend a container of charcoal be carried in the pocket for first aid when individuals are hiking in snake-infested woods.

Once swelling begins, the venom may not be able to transfer to the charcoal as easily as at first. As long as pain and swelling are being controlled by the compresses we would continue with this treatment and expect the venom was being attracted to the charcoal. If pain and swelling should progress, we would add ice packs to the extremity. Injections equivalent to 100 fatal doses of cobra venom had no poisonous effect when activated charcoal was added to a solution of the venom and shaken before injection into experimental animals.

CASE HISTORIES

While we do not recommend the exclusive use of charcoal in venomous snake bites until more experience is gained, because of the potential seriousness of the situation, the following instances of which we are aware indicate that charcoal certainly warrants consideration in the first aid treatment of such bites.

Our first case was reported to us by telephone.

A couple living in a remote area of Arkansas called in great distress to report that their 1 1/2 year old son had been bitten on the chest by a copperhead moccasin. This snake may cause death in a small child. They were 60 miles down a winding road from the nearest hospital. The fang marks were surrounded by some swelling and the child was in great pain. We instructed the couple to get to the emergency room as quickly as possible, and told them to apply charcoal poultices one after the other, every ten minutes until they got there. We were greatly relieved when they called several hours later to report that the child was doing quite well. In fact, by the time they had gotten to the hospital, the child was asleep, the swelling had gone down and the pain had obviously stopped. The physician administered the antivenin to be on the safe side, but told them that he didn't really believe it was necessary. The child had no ill effects.

We have heard of another venomous snake bite successfully treated with charcoal. A 50-year old woman who was reared in Germany where she learned of home remedies, treated a cotton-mouth moccasin bite with six hours of continuous charcoal soaks to the affected foot.

She took charcoal by mouth. After that she made a poultice of crushed cabbage leaves for overnight use, and slept fairly comfortably. The next day it was still swollen but not very painful. She continued daily charcoal soaks. The swelling was not entirely gone for about five weeks, but eventually she completely recovered. She did not use any antivenin.

SPIDER BITES

The brown recluse spider produces a bite that gives little or no pain at first. Within 24 hours a purplish-red blister develops at the site of the bite, and extensive tissue death occurs beneath the bite producing a very deep and angry ulceration extending down to the bone and often lasting for weeks or months. Since there is no antidote and no antivenin, the only treatment generally recognized medically is that of wide surgical 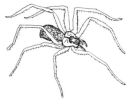 excision...or cutting away of flesh containing the venom, in the hope of physically removing all of the venom. This is a good treatment, but we have found that the treatment of choice for brown recluse spider bite is a compress of charcoal applied as soon after the bite as possible, preferably during the first 24 hours, with frequent changes.

CASE HISTORIES

We have had three experiences with brown recluse spider bites. The brown recluse, an innocent-appearing little creature, is extremely toxic. Its bite causes extensive tissue damage and finally necrosis (tissue death), with eventual sloughing of tissue, through skin, fascia, blood vessels, nerves, muscles and tendons, right down to the bone. It takes months to heal and leaves a deep, puckered scar.

Our first patient was a nurse, who recognized the spider and called for help. Charcoal poultices were applied and changed every 30 minutes through the night. The next morning, our hearts sank as we saw an angry, discolored, dime-sized blood blister at the site of the bite. But with prayer, we redoubled our efforts, and soon the swelling and discoloration began to subside. The following day it was decidedly better. The time intervals for changing the poultices was lengthened to 2 and then to 4 hours. After a week only a tiny, slightly red spot remained, which itched slightly; no slough occurred.

On hearing this case report, an anesthetist in one of our seminars related that just the previous day he had anesthetized a lady for the second time, to do a more extensive amputation of her foot that had been bitten over 2 months before! The first amputation had not removed all the damaged tissue, and it had failed to heal.

Our second case was not as fortunate as the nurse. She knew that she had been bitten, but did not recognize the nature of the creature. Two days had passed before we saw her, and the area around the bite was swollen, discolored, and quite uncomfortable. Nevertheless, vigorous applications of the poultices and soaking in charcoal water prevented serious damage, and she had only a minimal slough which healed in 2 weeks. Then she developed a tiny red, hemorrhagic rash (angiitis) on her leg, which cleared in five weeks. She continued to have swelling for over 6 months.

Our third case was a 60 year old man who called us from a Veterans Administration hospital. He had been bitten by a brown recluse spider two days before, having seen the spider and recognized it. He now had a large blood blister on his thumb just at the base, silver dollar size, with extensive swelling of the entire thumb and forefinger, with purplish discoloration of his whole hand. The VA surgeons offered him as the treatment of choice the removal of his thumb and the fleshy mound of muscle and bone at its base right back to the wrist in an attempt to save his hand. At that point he called us. We advised charcoal compresses changed every 30 minutes for the remaining 8 hours of the day, and every 2 hours during the night. Three months later, he drove over to show us the results of following our advice. He had a shallow, elastic scar which did not interfere at all with the movement of his thumb! The very fact he had a thumb would have caused the VA doctors to marvel.

Another case we know of, which had a single charcoal compress applied during the first eight hours, developed a superficial slough into the subcutaneous tissue, but healed in about three weeks.

EYE AND EAR CONDITIONS
TREATED WITH CHARCOAL

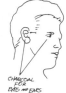
CHARCOAL
FOR
EYES AND EARS

The eyes are actually another lobe of the brain. A treatment of the eyes can result in a treatment to the brain, and it is well to remember that such afflictions of the brain as meningitis and encephalitis may respond somewhat to charcoal compresses and other treatment applied to the eyes.

Cellulitis of the face, eyelids, and ears can be effectively treated with a compress of charcoal. Earache (otitis media or otitis externa) can be treated by a charcoal compress molded over the exterior of the ear. A heat lamp, or a desk lamp with a 100 watt bulb, used over the compress to keep it warm, can increase its effectiveness in relieving pain. Cover the compress with kitchen plastic, or else continued moistening of the poultice under the lamp will be necessary, due to the drying effect of the lamp.

INFECTIONS

Activated charcoal can adsorb bacteria, viruses, and bacterial toxins. Charcoal has been reported to disinfect wounds, and to act as a deodorizer in various bodily ills.[37] Charcoal can be used for infected wound dressing

71

and for deodorizing. On the body surface charcoal will adsorb wound secretions, bacteria, carcinogens, toxins, products of allergies, and will reduce swelling by taking up excess tissue fluid and products of inflammation. Charcoal works better in an acid than in an alkaline medium. Charcoal has been used internally in Asiatic cholera, dysentery, diarrhea, and dyspepsia.[38]

Foot and mouth disease virus in a one percent suspension can be entirely adsorbed on charcoal when used in the amount of 10 grams of charcoal per 100cc of fluid (about two tablespoons per 1/2 cup). The virus is not destroyed but its activity is much reduced. Wood and coconut charcoal are less effective than bone charcoal for adsorbing foot and mouth disease virus. Sheep pox virus is adsorbed on bone charcoal effectively.

INTRAVENOUS CHARCOAL

Suspensions of colloidal charcoal (the water remaining after charcoal is stirred in and the black fraction allowed to settle) have been used intravenously in 100 veterinary cases of septicemia, metritis, mastitis, lymphangitis, and infected wounds. After the infusion of charcoal there was seen an increase in the number of neutrophils. Elevated body temperature returned to normal within one hour. The charcoal reportedly is filtered out in spleen, lymph nodes, liver, and other reticuloendothelial areas. Since patients receiving intravenous charcoal have sometimes experienced shortness of breath, it seems probable that capillaries in the lungs were irritated by the charcoal, at least temporarily. These patients were treated with intravenous injections of 0.001 grams per kilograms of body weight.[39] This interesting use of intravenous activated charcoal would seem to us to have very limited application, but under certain conditions might be lifesaving.

INFLAMMATION

We have seen pain in severe, throbbing and feverish cellulitis subside in a matter of five minutes after the application of a charcoal compress. The reaction is unbelievable unless actually observed. E.G. White once said, "One of the most beneficial remedies is pulverized charcoal...used in fomentations...the more severe inflammation of the eyes will be relieved by a poultice of charcoal, put in a bag, and dipped in hot or cold water as will best suit the case....If I could give this remedy some outlandish name, that no one knew but myself, it would have greater influence."[40]

COMMON DIGESTIVE PROBLEMS
(See also Chapter Seven)

The treatment of choice for food poisoning is charcoal. A dentist's young wife had just learned she had rheumatoid arthritis. She asked us to come by her husband's office to talk with them about dietary treatment for this condition. We arrived at 5:00 and were greeted at the door by the young lady with a most distressed look on her face. She complained of the sudden onset of extreme nausea. She, her dentist husband, along with the office receptionist, had eaten lunch together earlier in the day. The receptionist was just leaving by the back door complaining of the same sudden onset of discomfort, although not as severe as the dentist's wife. Retrieving charcoal from our car, we mixed a tablespoon in a large glass of water for the dentist's wife. Within ten minutes of drinking this concoction she was well. The receptionist refused the charcoal thinking her case not severe enough to warrant such "unsavory" treatment. However, her "mild" malady caused her to miss work the next day as she was still not well enough to venture out of her house.

A prominent Columbus, Georgia, executive was traveling in Mexico when he developed a bad case of tourista. He was having diarrhea 2-3 times an hour on the first day of his disease, with much discomfort in the abdomen. A Mexican doctor treated him with the usual antibiotics and Lomotil. He consulted his own doctor a

73

week later because the condition had settled down to 3-5 diarrheic stools a day with continuing discomfort. He got a change of medication but no change of symptoms. After 12 days of the disease and 8 medicines, he called us desperately seeking suggestions for a natural remedy. We began a routine of one tablespoon of charcoal in a glass of water, followed by a full glass of water every time he had a loose stool. Within two days he was entirely well...and sold on charcoal. Now he never travels without charcoal and takes a tablespoon with the first hint of a symptom.

Gas discomfort should be treated with charcoal as the best remedy. Abdominal pain will often subside within minutes after a tablespoon of charcoal.

BEAN GAS STUDY

A New York team of gastroenterologists compared three groups of people, one on placebo, one on simethicone (the standard drug treatment for gas), and the other on charcoal. They used breath hydrogen techniques to assess the amount of intestinal gas produced before and after treatment, and found activated charcoal to be quite superior.

The study was conducted by giving the ten healthy volunteers eight ounces of canned Heinz baked beans. They studied each subject on three occasions three days apart. Half an hour before the subject had the test meal, he was given four capsules of simethicone (80 mm), or 1.04 grams (less than one teaspoon) of activated charcoal, or a placebo. Half an hour after the test meal, each subject got a second dose of the same agent. The capsules were all identical in appearance and neither the subjects nor the physicians knew which agent was being used. For seven hours after the administration of the first dose, breath samples were analyzed for hydrogen content every 30 minutes, and abdominal discomfort and bloating scores were reported and recorded on a scale of zero to three in which zero represented none, one-mild, two-moderate, and three-severe. All ten volunteers had a rotation of the agents used. One subject turned out to be a non-producer of hydrogen and could not be scored objectively.

The charcoal significantly reduced breath hydrogen levels, bloating, and abdominal discomfort. Simethicone did not! The mean breath hydrogen level fell from 617 parts per million per hour with placebo to 178 parts per million per hour with activated charcoal. Simethicone was no better than placebo.

The number of subjects complaining of abdominal symptoms was reduced from seven with an average symptoms sum of eleven on placebo, to one person with a symptoms sum of one on activated charcoal![41]

SEVERE GASTROINTESTINAL
DISORDERS

The use of charcoal for milder gastrointestinal disorders, such as gas, nausea and vomiting, and diarrhea are so well known as to make it difficult to select a case history. In fact, we have come to believe that any diarrhea adequately treated with charcoal that does not respond, usually proves to be some very serious disorder, such as cancer or severe malabsorption. But the following two cases illustrate that it can be useful adjunctive therapy even in more serious abdominal conditions.Idiopathic

CHRONIC INTESTINAL
PSEUDO-OBSTRUCTION

This strange condition gives all the signs and symptoms of intestinal obstruction, but no organic cause for it has been found. Patients usually undergo repeated surgeries, and become malnourished and often die because of loss of electrolytes, etc.

Several years ago, a middle-aged lady came to our conditioning center "as a last resort." She had had abdominal surgery at least 12 times in the last five years, and was having to be admitted to the hospital every two or three weeks for gastric intubation and intravenous fluids. She was rapidly becoming debilitated. She was put on large amounts of activated charcoal by mouth, and fomentations to the abdomen several times a day. On the third day, she began to get abdominal distention and nausea. She was given a large dose of charcoal by mouth and a fomentation applied, which was afterward replaced by a large charcoal poultice to the abdomen.

The following morning, the distention was gone, and we rejoiced that she was hungry. The treatments were continued, and she was given a regular vegetarian diet. She never had another attack! She continues to use charcoal daily.

CHRONIC RELAPSING PANCREATITIS

A 26-year old woman came to the conditioning center, planning to stay for two or three months. She had had several abdominal operations in the past three years, and had finally been diagnosed as having chronic pancreatitis. Because of the severe unremitting pain and debility, her physicians were considering total removal of her pancreas. Hoping to find some relief short of this drastic procedure, her husband had his job transferred to our area so that she could be treated at our institute. They "knew" treatment would take several months. The patient was on potent medications for pain and nausea. Despite these, she was having continuous pain, nausea and vomiting. We asked if she were willing to stop her medications, which we felt were aggravating her condition. She reluctantly agreed.

She was put on fomentations to the abdomen, charcoal

by mouth, and large abdominal poultices at night. Because of the severity of her symptoms, her lifestyle counselor stayed in her room continually for the first 48 hours. The following day, the nausea was better, and she could retain liquids. She was rolled into the sun for a few minutes several times a day.

Day by day her pain declined, and her appetite improved. In two weeks she was taking long walks, and by three weeks was walking five to six miles a day. After four weeks, she was completely symptom-free, and they returned to their home, praising the Lord.

JAUNDICE IN THE NEWBORN

The need for exchange blood transfusion in babies with Rh incompatibility (erythroblastosis fetalis) has been cut in some places by more than seventy percent with the use of charcoal. If a bilirubin level in a newborn goes above ten milligrams, the infant should be given a teaspoon of charcoal stirred in sufficient water to pass through a nipple every two to three hours. Since serum bilirubin levels usually reach over twenty milligrams percent before an exchange transfusion begins to be considered, the charcoal regimen affords an earlier treatment and will often stabilize the bilirubin at much less than twenty milligrams.[42]

Breast feeding encourages the development of mild jaundice in the newborn, since a hormone in milk retards the processing of bilirubin by the liver. This small elevation of the serum bilirubin is not injurious to the baby, and probably stimulates development of the nervous system. Unless excessively high levels develop (over 25 mg/deciliter) an exchange transfusion is usually not considered.

The very first case of neonatal jaundice which we treated with charcoal was a breast fed baby who developed jaundice four days after birth. On his fifth day the baby was sent to a laboratory with his father where his total bilirubin level was 12 milligrams percent. Twelve hours later it was at 14.5 milligrams percent and was at 16 milligrams percent six hours after that. A consultant agreed with our suspicion of an ABO incompatibility. At this point we began six hour bilirubin determinations with appropriate associated laboratory tests. When the bilirubin rose to 18 milligrams percent the consultant began to prepare for an exchange transfusion. That same hour, upon our suggestion, the mother began administering as much charcoal solution as she could get the baby to accept, and sat in the sunlight with the baby undressed in her lap, giving over an hour of exposure to both front and back (babies can tolerate more sunlight before getting a sunburn than can adults). At the next six hour bilirubin check the level was down to 16.5 milligrams percent and we knew we had avoided the hazardous exchange transfusion. Continuing with this treatment the bilirubin began to clear and was down to 4 milligrams percent by the tenth day.

Since low oxygen rather than high bilirubin has been implicated in the cause of brain damage in these infants, every attempt should be made to keep a circulation of fresh air around the baby. If charcoal feeding is started at twelve hours of age it is less effective than when begun at four hours of age, as the enterohepatic circulation of bilirubin may play a critical role in determining the size of the bilirubin pool during first few hours of life.

LIVER AND KIDNEY FAILURE
Patients with liver and kidney failure can be treated sometimes even in the home with large compresses of

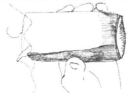

charcoal placed over the back or over the abdomen. Charcoal can also be given by mouth in an attempt to prevent toxins from building up in the blood.[43]

We have applied charcoal compresses to the back in kidney failure and observed the strong odor of urine on the compress the following morning after eight hours over night. Charcoal enemas may also be given.

A 44 year old nurse developed widespread metastases from a cancer of the colon. Her ureters became blocked partially by the cancer and her urinary wastes began to rise in her blood. Each week her blood urea nitrogen

(BUN) was about 5 milligrams higher than the week before. When the level reached 130, we began charcoal compresses each night and charcoal by mouth (1 tablespoon every 4 hours) during the day. The next week her BUN was down 5 mg. and continued to fall about 5 mg. per week until her death from the cancer.

During her last few weeks the nausea and abdominal discomfort she had experienced because of the extremely high BUN was much relieved and finally stopped when her BUN fell below 100 mg.

Abdominal pain, treated with a compress of activated charcoal, laying it over the entire abdomen and sides often gives great relief of pain in a short time. The pain of sore throat, earache, sprains, arthritis, pleurisy, and other pains should be given a trial of a charcoal compress. Often the pain that has gone unabated for hours will be relieved in a matter of ten minutes.

The gastrointestinal tract is one of the most important systems for the removal of toxins, the lungs, skin, and urinary systems being other routes of excretion of toxins. As materials are secreted from the blood into the gastrointestinal tract, the toxins may be either digested or reabsorbed into the blood stream. If charcoal is present in the gastrointestinal tract, the toxic substances may adsorb onto the charcoal. Since toxins may be actively secreted into the gastrointestinal tract from the bloodstream, charcoal can effectively cleanse the blood when taken orally.

Fiber from fruits, vegetables, and whole grains also act as material to adsorb toxins. Many cancer producing chemicals leave the body in this manner. It is likely that one of the reasons vegetarians have less cancer than others is that cancer producing substances which have found their way into the bloodstream, by inhalation, by ingestion or via the skin, can be secreted into the intestinal tract from the blood, and there be taken up by vegetable fiber and complex carbohydrates. The toxic substances are then rendered harmless and can be eliminated from the intestines with the wastes.

ENDOMETRITIS AFTER
ABORTION OR CHILDBIRTH

Back in 1930, Nahmacher in Germany treated septic endometritis following criminal abortions with installation of charcoal into the uterine cavity. He would make charcoal pencils, introducing them into the uterus through the cervix. Toxins and bacteria were adsorbed onto the charcoal. He reported raging fevers to subside in a few hours. Once he started using the intrauterine charcoal, he never lost another case of septic abortion. He reported almost immediate cessation of malodorous discharges in infected abortions treated with charcoal.

He also reported that fever after the birth of a baby was very favorably influenced by intrauterine charcoal therapy. As soon as a foul smelling discharge and low grade fever began, the patients were treated with five to six days of raising the head of the bed to promote drainage, an ice bag applied to the pelvis, and charcoal installations into the uterus. In all cases a reduction in temperature occurred the day following and was normal

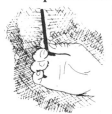

by the second day. The odor disappeared at once. In over 90 percent of the cases it was unnecessary to insert charcoal pencils more than once.

His method of making the charcoal pencils is interesting. He heated water, charcoal and starch together until thickened. After slight cooling, he poured strips of the tacky material onto a greased pan. When completely congealed, he placed them in a barely warm oven overnight to dry. He could then pick them up if he handled them gently.

WHITENING THE TEETH

For polishing and cleaning the teeth, there is nothing superior to charcoal. It has been used by dentists for years and can be used just as easily in the home. Simply dip a moistened soft bristled toothbrush in charcoal. With a jiggling motion or small round polishing circles, brush the teeth. Rinse well. Use dental floss to remove any tiny bits of charcoal from between your teeth where you may have fillings, or brush again with a soft bristled toothbrush using a little tooth paste. You will have the best cleaned teeth possible. For badly stained teeth, more frequent brushings with charcoal may be needed. It should not be used daily, however, over a period of years since no studies have been done to test abrasiveness.

POISON IVY

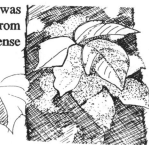

A 38 year old sergeant was given a medical discharge from the Army because of an intense sensitivity to poison ivy. His sensitivity was so severe that one particular bout with the problem had resulted in a painful 5-week stay at Ft. Benning's Martin Army Hospital complete with IV fluids, cortisone and a struggle just getting back to normal.

His wife called us early one morning asking us if we would see her husband. He had taken a walk in the country the day before and now his hands, feet, face and other areas were swollen tight. His eyelids were swollen shut and fingers were so stiff he could not bend them. We were reluctant to treat him as they insisted--without hospitalization and with simpler remedies than cortisone (which gave him wildly distressing thoughts). When we saw him he was feeling faint and nauseated. We showed his wife how to make charcoal compresses and instructed her on how to mix charcoal for oral administration. With these treatments he gradually improved during the day and could open his eyes by the next morning and close his fingers enough to grasp a steering wheel. After five days, he was entirely well. We were all impressed.

CHARCOAL AND CHOLESTEROL

STUDY FOUND CHARCOAL EFFECTIVE IN LOWERING CHOLESTEROL LEVELS

Activated charcoal has been found to lower the concentration of total lipids, cholesterol and triglycerides in the blood serum, liver, heart and brain. A study reported by the British journal *Lancet,* found that patients with high blood cholesterol levels were able to reduce total cholesterol 25%. Not only that, but while LDL (the "bad" cholesterol) was lowered as much as 41%, HDL (the "good" kind) /LDL cholesterol ratio was doubled! The patients took the equivalent of roughly one quarter ounce (approximately 1 tablespoon) of activated charcoal three times daily. Another study conducted by the National Institute of Public Health in Finland, suggested that activated charcoal was as effective in reducing high cholesterol levels as the drug, lovastatin. More studies are needed in this area, but even if the charcoal therapy is not as effective, it certainly would be considerably less expensive, while possessing none of the dangerous side effects of the drug. Our own experience has been that charcoal is a valuable part of a total cholesterol reducing program, but that long-term lifestyle changes must be maintained to permanently reduce high cholesterol.

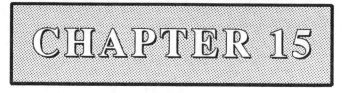

CHAPTER 15

WHAT IS THE PROBLEM?

Poisoning?

Go to... 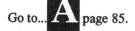 page 85.

Bee sting, snake, spider, fire ant, etc. bite?

Go to... **B** page 87.

You don't know?

Quickly read the next few paragraphs to help in identifying just what the problem may be...

MIGHT IT BE A BITE OR STING?

If your child is crying for no obvious reason, check all over the body for localized swelling, extreme tenderness and redness. Also look for puncture wounds, stingers or the presence of an afflicting creature. If this seems to be the problem, go to... **B**, page 87.

POISONING CAN BE SUSPECTED IF:
* the child has been exploring under the sinks
* any medicine bottles are open
* anything is out of place in the house or garage
* anyone in the household is taking medications:
    - pain killers
    - tranquilizers
    - antidepressants
    - Lomotil
    - medication for bedwetting
    - iron tablets in pregnancy.
* alcohol or recreational drugs left unattended

Also, if your child is exhibiting any of the following symptoms, you may further assume poisoning.

* has suddenly become ill
* is uncharacteristically lethargic
* is pale, weak, short of breath
* appears to be losing consciousness
* is acting confused or having seizures
* can no longer walk normally
* has blue lips or fingernails
* has burns in the mouth or throat
* is vomiting or having severe abdominal pains

If you now suspect poisoning, go to... **A** page 85.

If you are still not sure...

COULD THERE BE ANOTHER CAUSE OF SICKNESS?

* Any signs of infectious diseases such as:
                    - fever
                    - sore throat
                    - earache
* Is anyone else in the family ill?
* Has the child fallen or had an accident (check especially the head)
* Is an epileptic seizure possible?
* In warm weather, might the child be having sun stroke or heat exhaustion?
* Is there bruising or bleeding?
* Has there been recent emotional stress:
                    - attempted suicide
                    - death of family member
                    - divorce
* Does the child take insulin or any other kind of medication such as for heart or lung disease?

If this seems to be the case, child (or adult) should be properly cared for by appropriate personnel.

If it is known that a child took a certain medication, try to determine:

- the maximum quantity possibly taken;
- exactly when it might have been taken;
- how many pills were in the bottle and how many now remain?
- how much is left of a container of liquid and how much was there in the beginning?
- when was the child last seen before being left unattended?

Symptoms are slow to appear sometimes if only a small amount of the poison has been swallowed. If a child has swallowed a small amount of kerosene and hasn't started to cough, choke or gag within 20-30 minutes, it is unlikely that there will be any respiratory problems.

A POISONING: WHAT TO DO

- **Say a prayer** for wisdom, speed and calmness.
- **Manually induce vomiting** by massaging the back of the throat with a finger unless gasoline, kerosene, lighter fluid or a caustic or acid has been swallowed. If that is the case:

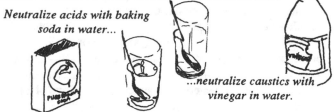

Neutralize acids with baking soda in water...

...neutralize caustics with vinegar in water.

- **Administer charcoal**
- If the charcoal can be swallowed before the child becomes lethargic or in danger of being unable to swallow, much is gained.
- Don't use a large amount of water to stir the charcoal into, put a straw into it and suck it way back on the tongue and swallow quickly.
- It is quite likely that this will be the only treatment the child will need.

Estimated amount of poison or medicine taken	Charcoal to be used if person has **not** eaten in last 2 hrs	Charcoal to be used if person has eaten in last 2 hrs.
1 teaspoon 1-2 tablets, 1-2 capsules	1-2 T stirred in water. Drink this plus 2 more glasses of water	4-10 T stirred in water. Drink this plus 2 more glasses of water
1 tablespoon, 3-5 tablets, 2-5 capsules	3-4 T powder administered same as above	6-15 T powder administered same as above
Unknown	1-5 T powder administered same as above	5-15 T powder administered same as above

Repeat all doseages in 10 minutes, or if symptoms begin to worsen.

A small child will struggle vigorously and will need to be held down. A spoon or ideally a small bulb syringe can be used to transfer a small amount of the charcoal solution into the mouth. The child should be held in a position making swallowing the only option, preferably on the back. Then another small amount put into the mouth until the charcoal is all gone. (**Caution: Do not put anything in a child's mouth if sleepy, fainting or otherwise unable to swallow. In such cases, prompt professional attention is vital.**) The charcoal can be repeated as often as needed. Give plenty of water subsequently to insure easier passage of the charcoal.

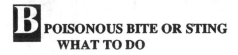

POISONOUS BITE OR STING
WHAT TO DO

BEE STING

1. Immediate Relief

 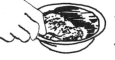 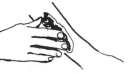

One part charcoal + *Enough water = Smear on sting*
to make paste

2.

For multiple stings
(As common with yellow jackets)

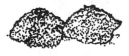

2 cups charcoal + *Bathtub of water*

3.

For long term relief, place a charcoal compress over the
sting site. (See the next page for instructions on how to
make a charcoal compress.)

MAKING A CHARCOAL COMPRESS

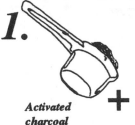

1.

Activated charcoal

+

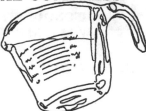

Enough water to make a paste - don't start with too much water.

2.

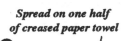

Spread on one half of creased paper towel

Fold other half over the charcoal paste

3.

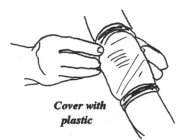

Position over afflicted area

Cover with plastic

1. Plastic keeps compress moist.

2. Change often depending on severity of bite.

3. A hospital tuck, a piece of sheet, or most porous materials can be used in place of paper towel.

4. It would be good to fold edges of compress over and tape to prevent charcoal from falling out.

5. Compresses can be made ahead of time and frozen for emergencies.

6. Flax seed or corn starch can be used with charcoal (1 to 1) to hold moisture for long term compresses.

TYPE OF PROBLEM	Ant, Mosquito, Chiggar bite (Page 92)	Bee sting (Page 89)	Multiple Bee Stings (Page 89)	Spider Bite (Page 92)	Snake Bite (Page 93)
INITIAL TREATMENT OF CHOICE	Charcoal Bandaid (See page 92)	Charcoal paste applied to sting area (See page 89.)	30 minute charcoal bath (See page 89)	Charcoal soak (See page 93) followed by...	1. Wash bite area 2. 1/2 hour cool charcoal soak 3. Compress to entire area 4. Drink 2T charcoal every 2 hrs for 6 hrs then 1 t every 4 hours for 24 hrs
ADDITIONAL TREATMENTS		Charcoal compress (See page 90)	Charcoal compresses	Charcoal Compress	
DURATION OF TREATMENTS	Until irritation ceases Change when dry	Change every 10 min. for 1 hr then leave one on for at least 8 hours or until swelling and pain are gone	Change every 10 minutes for 1 hour then leave one on for at least 8 hours.	Change every 30 minutes for 8 hours then every 2 hours for 8 hours then every 2-4 hours until healing is complete	Change compress every 10-15 min. until swelling and pain are gone. Add ice packs if pain and swelling persist.

This chart is a summary of the information found in Chapter 15, section B. For acute bee sting reactions or snake bites, it is always advisable, if possible, to summon professional medical help. However, you cannot use too much charcoal as a first aid treatment. Also, time is of the essence in these cases.

ANT, MOSQUITO, CHIGGAR BITES

1.

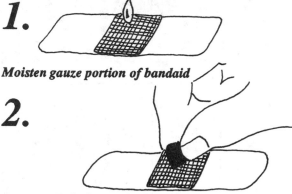

Moisten gauze portion of bandaid

2.

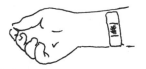

*Rub charcoal tablet or sprinkle charcoal
on gauze till well blackened*

3.

Place bandaid over bitten area

SPIDER BITES

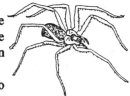

- A charcoal compress should be applied as soon as possible. (See previous page for instructions in making a charcoal compress.)

- Soaking in charcoal water is also effective.

- Change compress often, preferably every 30 minutes for a brown recluse spider bite, for the first eight (8) hours, then every two (2) hours for the next eight (8) hours. Thereafter the charcoal compress should be changed every two (2) to eight (8) hours until healing is accomplished.

SNAKE BITES

- Swelling and pain are evidences of envenomation in a snakebite.
- The swelling should be in evidence within ten minutes of being bitten or one should question whether there has been envenomation. If there has been:

1.

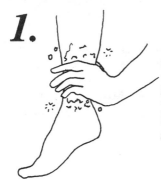

For venomous bites (or poison ivy), immediately wash the area well with soap and water, or flood with a solution of charcoal.

2.

Venomous bites may be submerged in cool charcoal water for an hour and followed by a compress. Use 1/2 cup of charcoal to about 2-5 gallons of water.

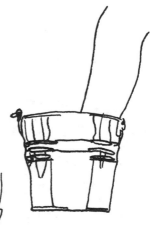

3.

Apply a large charcoal compress covering almost the entire bitten extremity, centering over the bite.

- Once swelling begins the venom may not be able to transfer to the charcoal as easily as at first.

- Change compress over the immediate vicinity of the snakebite every ten to fifteen minutes.

- Take approximately two tablespoonsful of activated charcoal by mouth every two hours for three doses, and one teaspoonful every four hours for the next 24 hours. Each dose should be followed by two glasses of water.

- The sooner charcoal is applied, the more effective the treatment should be.

- As long as pain and swelling are being controlled by the compresses, continue with this treatment and expect that the venom is being attracted to the charcoal.

- If pain and swelling should progress, add ice packs to the extremity and get to a hospital emergency room as quickly as possible,

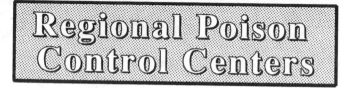

Regional Poison Control Centers

ALABAMA
Alabama Poison Center
809 University Blvd., East
Tuscaloosa; AL 35401
205-345-0600
800-462-0800

ARIZONA
Arizona Poison and Drug
Information Center
AZ Health Sciences Center,
Room 3204K
University of Arizona
Tucson, AZ 85724
602-626-6016
(800-362-0101-Arizona)

CALIFORNIA
University of California
Davis Medical Center
Regional Poison Center, 2315
Stockton Blvd.
Sacramento, CA 95817
916-453-3692
800-852-7221(N. California)

Los Angeles County
Medical Association
Regional Poison Information
Center 1925 Wilshire Blvd
Los Angeles, CA 90057
213-484-5151

San Diego Regional
Poison Center
University of California
Medical Center
225 Dickinson St., H925
San Diego, CA 92103
619-294-6000

San Francisco Bay Area
Regional Poison Center
1E86, SF General Hospital
1001 Potrero Avenue
San Francisco, CA 94110
415-476-6600
800-233-3360

COLORADO
Rocky Mt. Poison Center
645 Bannock St.
Denver, CO 80204
303-893-7774
800-525-5042 (Montana)
800-442-2701 (Wyoming)
800-332-3073 (Colorado)

DISTRICT OF COLUMBIA
(Washington, D.C.)
National Capitol Poison Center
Georgetown Univ. Hospital
3800 Reservoir Road, NW
Washington, DC 20007
202-625-3333

GEORGIA
Georgia Poison Control Center
Grady Memorial Hospital
Box 26066/80 Butler St. SE
Atlanta, GA 30335
404-589-4400
800-282-5846 (Georgia)

FLORIDA
Tampa Bay Regional Poison
Control Center
P.O. Box 18582
Tampa, FL 33679
813-253-4444
800-282-3171

ILLINOIS
Central & Southern Illinois
Poison Resource Center
800 E. Carpenter St.
Springfield, IL 62769
217-753-3330
(800-252-2022-Illinois)

INDIANA
Indiana Poison Center
Wishard Memorial Hospital
1001 W. Tenth Street
Indianapolis, IN 46202
317-630-7351
(800-382-9097-Indiana)

IOWA
University of Iowa
Hospitals and Clinics
Poison Control Center
Pharmacy Department
Iowa City, IA 52242
319-356-2922
800-272-6477

KENTUCKY
Kentucky Regional Poison
Center of Kosair
Children's Hospital
P.O. Box 35070
Louisville, KY 40232
502-589-8222
(800-722-5725-Kentucky)

LOUISIANA
Louisiana Regional Poison
Control Center
1501 Kings Highway
Shreveport, LA 71130
318-425-1524
800-535-0525

MARYLAND
Maryland Poison Center
120 N. Pine Street Center
Baltimore, MD 21201
301-528-7701
800-492-2414 (Maryland)

MICHIGAN
Poison Control Center
Children's Hospital of
Michigan (313-494-5711)
3901 Beaubien Blvd.
Detroit, MI 48201
800-572-1655 (Northern or
    Western Michigan)
800-462-6642
    (Southeastern Michigan)
Blodgett Regional Poison
Center
1840 Wealthy Street, SE
Grand Rapids, MI 49506
616-774-7854
800-632-2727 (Michigan)

MINNESOTA
Hennepin Poison Center
701 Park
Minneapolis, MN 55415
612-347-3141
Minnesota Poison Control
System 612-221-2113
640 Jackson St.
St. Paul, MN 55101
800-222-1222

MISSOURI
Cardinal Glennon Children's
Hospital
1465 S. Grand Avenue
St. Louis, MO 63104
314-772-5200
800-392-9111 (Missouri)

NEBRASKA
Mid-Plains Poison Control
Center (402-390-5400)
Children's Memorial
Hospital 800-642-9999
(Nebraska)
8301 Dodge Street
Omaha, NB 68114
(States surrounding
Nebraska) 800-228-9515

NEW JERSEY
New Jersey Poison
    Information and
    Education System
201 Lyons Avenue
Newark, NJ 07112
201-296-8005
(800-962-1253)

NEW MEXICO
New Mexico Poison and
Drug Information Center
University of New Mexico
Albuquerque, NM 87131
505-843-2551
800-432-6866 (New
Mexico)

NEW YORK
New York City
Poison Center
455 First Avenue,
Room 123
New York, NY 10016
212-340-4494
212-764-7667

Nassau County Medical
Center Long Island Regional
Poison Control Center
2201 Hempstead Turnpike
East Meadow, NY 11554
516-542-2323

NORTH CAROLINA
Duke Poison Control Center
Box 3007
Duke University
    Medical Center
Durham, NC 27710
919-684-8111
800-672-1697

OHIO
Central Ohio Poison Control
Center 614-228-1323
700 Children's Drive
Columbus, OH 43205
800-682-7625
Southwest Ohio Regional
    Poison Control
System, Drug & Poison
Information Center
University of Cincinnati,
College of Medicine
231 Bethesda Avenue ML
144 Cincinnati, OH 45267
513-872-5111
800-872-5111

PENNSYLVANIA
Pittsburgh Poison Center
125 DeSoto Street
Pittsburgh, PA 15213
412-647-5600

UTAH
Intermountain Regional
Poison Control Center
50 N. Medical Drive
Bldg. 428
Salt Lake City, UT 84132
800-662-0062 (Utah)
801-581-2151
801-581-2973 (deaf only)

WASHINGTON
Seattle Poison Center
Children's Orthopedic
Hospital and Medical
Center, Box 5371
4800 Sand Point Way, NE
Seattle, WA 98105
206-526-2121
800-732-7985

INDEX

Gag, 28, 30, 32
Gas, 5, 42, **76, 77**
Gastritis, 5
Gastrointestinal dialysis, 49
Gastrointestinal disorders, 49, 51, 77, 81
Golden seal, 54

Haydon, Dr. Frank, 47
Healing
   Physiological, 2, 3
   Psychological, 2
Herbicides, 37
Homeopathic pharmacopoeia, 5
Homeopathic physicians, 5
Hemoperfusion, 36, 42
Hops, 15

Ileostomy, 12, 46
Infections, 73
Intestinal pseudo-obstruction, 77, 78
Intravenous, 74
Ipecac
   cartagena root, 19
   compared with charcoal, 18, 24
   emetine, 19, 20
   narcotic, 17
   slow acting, 17, 18
   vomiting, 17, 19, 20, 37
Infections, 11, 15, **73**
Inflammation, 74
Interference with nutrients, **59-61**
Iron intoxication, 57

JAMA, 60
Jaundice of newborn, 79, 80
Journal of Applied Toxicology, 54

Kidney failure, 80
Kilns, 7

Lantana poisoning, 54
Lavage, 20
Linden, 50
Liver failure, 80
Lomotil, 75

Malathion, 23
Meningitis, 73
Microdialysis, 38, **49**, 51
Milk, 22, 79
Milk of Magnesia, 63
Mucomyst, 25, 37
Mushrooms, **35, 36**

Nahmacher, 82
Nasogastric tube, 50
Nausea, 40
Neonatal jaundice, 79
Nervous indigestion, 5
Nutrient interference, **59-61**
North American Indians, 5

Odors, 3, 11, 12, 33, **45-48**, 73, 80, 82
Okinawa, 53
Orthopedic casts, 46, **47**
Otitis external, 73
Otitis media, 73
Overdoses, 17, 36

Pancreatitis, 78, 79
Pediatricians, 17
Phenobarbital, 49, 50

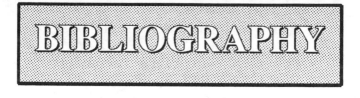

BIBLIOGRAPHY

1. **Physician's Desk Reference** (PDR), 39th ed., p. 1748, 1985.
2. DiSalvo PhD, R.M. Ancient Remedy? **Science News** 119:3, 1981.
3. Earl, D.E. *Charcoal: Andre' Mayer Fellowship Report*, HD:9559. C44 E27 Auburn Library.
4. **Acta Pharmacologica et Toxicologica,** 4:275, 1948.
5. **Archives of Environmental Health** 1:512, December, 1960.
6. Cooney, David O., **Activated Charcoal.** New York: Marcel Dekker, Inc. 1980, p.4.
7. Curtis, R.A. and J. Barone, et al. *Efficacy of Ipecac and Activated Charcoal/Cathartic.* **Archives of Internal Medicine** 144:48-52, 1984.
8. **International Medical News Service** quoting Lovejoy, F. H. *Encourage Parents to Keep Ipecac Syrup in House.* **Pediatric News** 18:39, 1984.
9. Wauters, J.P. and C. Rossel, et al. *Amanita phalloides Poisoning Treated by Early Charcoal Hemoperfusion.* **British Medical Journal,** November 25, 1978, p. 1465. (comment by Dr. H.R. Brunner).
10. **Archives of Internal Medicine** 145:44 January 1985

11. Sintek, C. and L. Hendeles, et al. *Inhibition of Theophylline Absorption by Activated Charcoal.* **The Journal of Pediatrics,** 94:314- 316, 1979.

12. Radomski, L. and G.D. Park, et al. *Model for Theophylline Overdose Treatment with Oral Activated Charcoal.* **Clinical Pharmacol. Ther.** March, 1984, p. 402-408.

13. Ravaut, P. *Pulverized Wood Charcoal in Prophylaxis and Treatment of Diarrhea in the Field.* **Presse Medicale,** Paris March 25, 1915 page 101.

14. Kelemen, G. *Efficacy of Charcoal in Catarrh of Gastrointestinal Tract.* **Muenchener Medizinische Woshenschrift,** [658](Nr.40):1378, October 5, 1915.

15. **Journal of the American Medical Association** 64:1882,May 29, 1915.

16. **AMA Archives of Industrial Health,** 18:511-520, December, 1958.

17. Von Haam, E. and H.L. Titus, et al. *Effect of Carbon Blacks on Carcinogenic Compounds.* **Proceedings of the Society For Experimental Biology and Medicine** 98:95-98, 1958.

18. **Vaschebnoe Delo** (Kiev) (4):79-84, April 1984.

19. Chamuleau, R.A.F.M. and A. Dupont, et al. *Activated Charcoal and Ammonium Production.* **The Lancet** p. 633-634, September 19, 1981.

20. **Emergency Medicine** September 30,1985.

21. **Orthopaedic Review** Volume 12[5]:127, May 1983.

22. Muck, O. *Behavior of Animal Charcoal in Respect to Lesion Caused by Bacillus Pyocyaneus.* **Muenchener Medizinische Wochenschrift** No. 6 p. 297, February 8, 1910.

23. Csillag, J. *Animal Charcoal in the Treatment of Eczema.* **Dermatologische Wochenschrift** 95:1328-1329, 1932.

24. Beckett, R., et al. *Charcoal Cloth and Malodorous Wounds.* **The Lancet** p. 594, September 13, 1980.

25. **New England Journal of Medicine** 307:642-644, 1982 and **Clinical Pharmacol. Ther.**, 33: 351-354, 1983 and J. Pediatr. 102:474-476, 1983

26. **The Lancet** 1981;2:117-8

27. Levy, G. *Gastrointestinal Clearance of Drugs with Activated Charcoal.* **New England Journal of Medicine** 307:676-678, 1982.

28. Dupuis, Robert E. & Slaghter, Richard L. *Severe Theophylline Toxicity.* **American Journal of Medicine**, 1984

29. Pass, M.A., et al. *Administration of Activated Charcoal for the Treatment of Lantana Poisoning of Sheep and Cattle.* **Journal of Applied Toxicology** 4[5]:267-9, 1984.

30. Spyker, D.A. *Activated Charcoal Reborn - Progress in Poison Management.* **Archives of Internal Medicine** 145:43-44, January 1985.

31. **Journal of Animal Science** 34:322-325, February 1972.

32. **Activated Charcoal**, Cooney, David O., New York: Marcel Dekker, Inc. page 63, 1980.

33. Dietzel: **Atoth. Ztg.** 47:283, 1932
34. **Bulletin de la Société de Chime Biologique** 27:513-518, October-December, 1945.
35. **Bulletin de la Société scientifique d'hygiene alimentaire et d'alimentation rationnelle de l'homme.** 36:114-121; 1948.
36. Chung, D.C. and J.E. Murphy, et al. *In-Vivo Comparison of the Adsorption Capacity of "Superactive Charcoal" and Fructose with Activated Charcoal and Fructose.* **Journal of Toxicology-Clinical Toxicology** 19[2]:219-225, 1982.
37. **JAMA** 64:1671,1915
38. **Quarterly Journal of Pharmacology** 1:334-337, July-September 1928
39. David O. Cooney. **Activated Charcoal.** New York: Marseille Dekker, Inc. 1980 page 123
40. E.G. White **Selected Messages Volume 2**, Washington D.C., Review and Herald Publishing Association page 294 1958
41. Hill, Thomas, *Charcoal Works Best to Control Intestinal Gas.* **The Medical Post**, December 24, 1985, p. 6.
42. **Medical World News**, February 17, 1967
43. **The Lancet** 1:1301, 1974